botanical
beauty

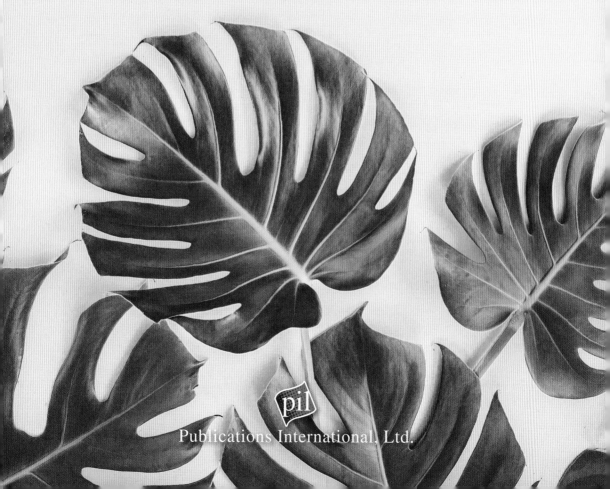

pil

Publications International, Ltd.

Let's get social!

@Publications_International

@PublicationsInternational

www.pilbooks.com

Table of Contents

Chapter 1

THINKING ABOUT YOUR SKIN

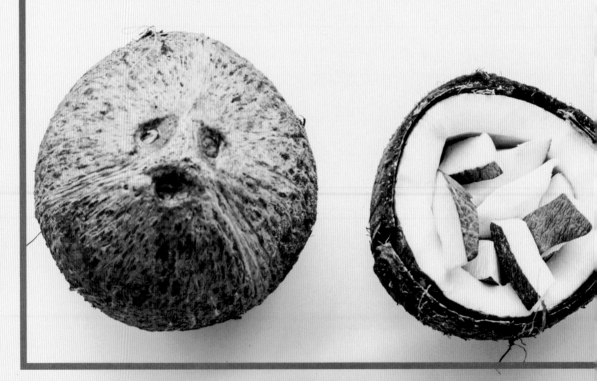

It's time to think about your skin
. . . and skin conditions.

The reason why treatments for skin conditions are so plentiful is because skin ailments, although usually minor as far as health risk is concerned, are so common. But skin conditions are also visible, uncomfortable, and demand attention.

Over time, useless natural remedies for the skin were smoothly weeded out—many were topical remedies, so it was usually obvious whether they worked or not. People kept the skin remedies that worked effectively and incorporated them into tradition. Luckily, plentiful skin treatments exist today.

To get started, familiarize yourself with a rich variety of herbs, oils, poultices, and other skin care remedies. Then, learn about how to apply these remedies to a host of skin conditions.

But first, let's learn about the healing powers of coconut, a substance that's used in a myriad of cultures throughout the world.

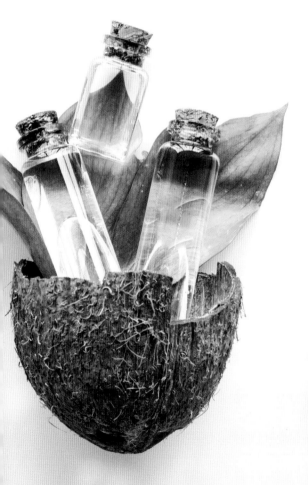

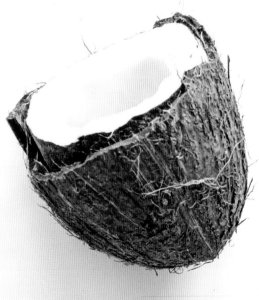

Not only can people consume the goodness of the coconut, people can wear coconuts, too—on their face and body, that is! Coconuts have been extolled for their radiant properties in beauty and personal care. Coconut oil may be one of the best skin creams, hydrating serums, and moisturizing lotions available. The unique properties of coconuts make them extremely versatile and useful for a myriad of beauty and hygienic habits.

The cell membranes in the skin are made up of three fat-containing substances: glycolipids (lipids with a carbohydrate component that helps to identify cells), phospholipids (lipids with a phosphate component that provide structure and function to cells), and cholesterol (the substance that is found in all cells of the body).

Phospholipids, made of saturated and unsaturated fatty acids, are the largest component of cell membranes. The balance of these three fatty acids is important for proper cell function and it is critical to human and animal health. The fatty acids in coconuts contribute to a healthy balance of these fatty acids in the cell membranes of the skin.

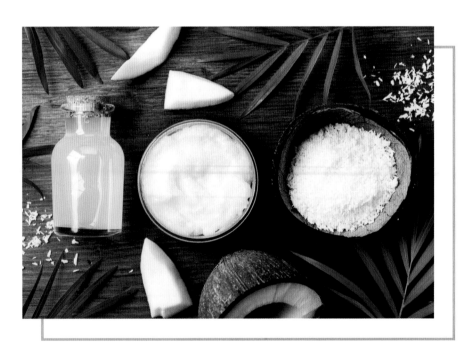

Aging, heat and cold, medications, skin treatments, and the sun can affect the hydration of the skin in a multitude of ways. Replacing this hydration can be done both externally and internally.

Proper hydration is essential for the skin's cell membranes. The surface skin cells do not dry out as fast or as much and the dead skin cells are reduced or are easily eliminated. As a result, the skin's pores do not get as clogged with dirt and impurities and excess oils do not accumulate, which also reduces the possibility of acne and infections.

Coconut oil provides hydration and essential fatty acids for healthy skin along with proper skin care. Coconut oil helps to protect the skin from free radicals and their aging effects and may help to improve the skin's appearance with its anti-aging benefits. Coconut oil acts as an antioxidant since it is stable, resists oxidation, and contributes some vitamin E, an antioxidant vitamin.

When coconut oil is absorbed into the skin and connective tissues, it may help to reduce the appearance of fine lines and wrinkles. It accomplishes this by supporting the strength and suppleness of connective tissues. It also aids in the exfoliation of the outer layer of dead skin cells, which makes the skin look smoother. Plus, it has a delightful aroma that bathes the skin to the enjoyment of the wearer and those in the immediate vicinity.

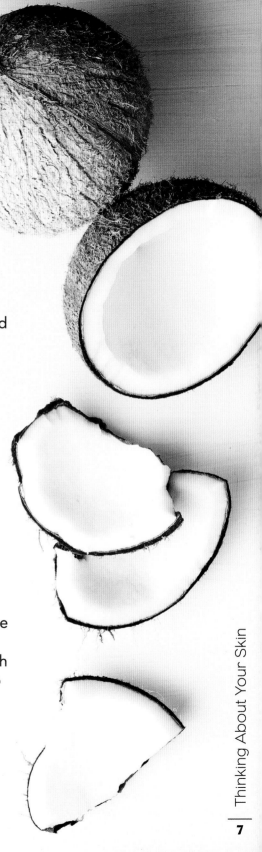

Thinking About Your Skin

Skin-Enhancing Qualities of Coconut Oil

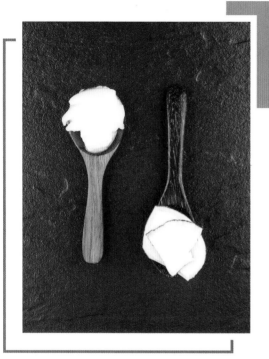

Several of the skin-enhancing qualities of coconut oil and coconut products include:

Acne relief: Coconut oil helps to keep skin hydrated and the pores open to reduce impurities and acne-related skin conditions.

Age spot minimizer: Coconut oil may diminish the look of age spots when used on a regular basis. It may accomplish this by keeping the area of the age spots and also the skin around the age spots supple.

Anti-aging defense: By smoothing the look of wrinkled skin, coconut oil may help to make skin appear younger. Younger skin does have more moisture that may dissipate over the years.

Baby lotion/massage oil: Warmed coconut oil with essential oil such as lavender, mint, rosemary or vanilla help to provide a relaxing, rejuvenating massage.

Bath/body moisturizer: Scented (or unscented) coconut massage oil can be applied to the skin both in and out of the bath or shower.

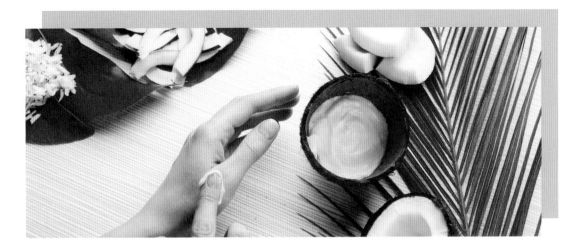

Body balm: Coconut-oil-based body balm is dense, hydrates, and repairs. It is similar to a lotion with light consistency that moistures but does not repair and a cream that is usually thicker, but is formulated for the face.

Bruise reducer: Coconut oil may not directly reduce the appearance of bruises, but similar to its effects on scars, sores, and stretch marks, it may promote the healing of the surrounding skin over time.

Cold sore reliever: Cold sores, often due to viruses, may benefit from coconut oil's anti-viral properties due to its composition of lauric and stearic fatty acids.

Deodorant: Coconut oil mixed with arrowroot powder, baking soda, cornstarch and scented or unscented essential oils can be used as a natural deodorant.

Diaper rash relief: Unless there is a known sensitivity to coconuts, a thin layer of coconut oil may provide some relief for chafed skin.

Facial mask: The antioxidants and fatty acids in coconut oil help to lubricate, smooth, and soften the skin when it is mixed with baking soda, lemon, turmeric, or yogurt as a facial mask.

Insect Repellent: The use of dodecanoic acid (DDA) against ticks has been validated and DDA is patented. The active ingredient DDA is a naturally occurring carboxylic acid, which is the broader classification of the acids that are found in coconut oil. Coconut oil has also been shown to show some repellency against mosquitos.

Lip balm: Coconut oil is a remedy for chapped lips since it is·semisolid at room temperature and can easily be spread by fingertips. Coconut balm is particularly soothing for the lips. A touch of natural extract, such as vanilla, gives coconut lip balm a tropical flavor.

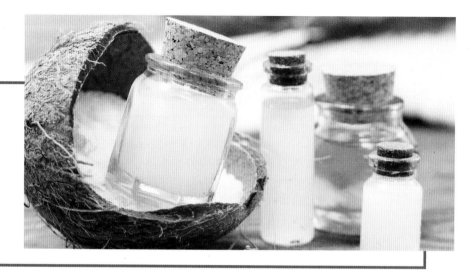

Massage Oil: The type of massage oil that one chooses may either enliven or soothe the body depending upon its consistency and aroma. Coconut oil provides lubrication and moisturizing for kneading, rubbing, and relaxing the body.

Simply blend one cup of coconut oil with a few drops of essential oils of choice, such as sweet and fragrant orange, geranium, rose, vanilla or ylang-ylang, or spicy and invigorating bergamot, cypress, fennel, frankincense, helichrysyum, lavender, myrrh, lemon grass, or rosemary.

Night cream: Apply coconut oil at night for its maximum moisturizing benefits, particularly around fine lines or wrinkles. A little left on the pillow at night will also moisturize the hair.

Nose Bleed Prevention: Coconut oil may be used to prevent nosebleeds that are attributed to dry nostrils from air pollutants, allergies, or extremes in temperature or humidity.

A little coconut oil that is dabbed onto the base of the nostrils may help to soften them and prevent cracking or drying.

Skin protection (dishpan hands, eczema, psoriasis): Coconut oil and coconut balm offer relief from allergic and chronic skin conditions that can be heightened by over-exposure to chemicals, sun, water and other skin-damaging factors.

Stretch mark/scar reducer: Pregnant women and people with minor scrapes and scratches can use coconut oil as a topical treatment for marks and scars. Coconut oil probably will not directly cause fading, but it may help to prevent dark spots and/or blisters from forming. Coconut oil may also help the surrounding skin retain its moisture and healthy glow.

Sun block/soother: Consuming coconuts and applying coconut oil to the skin may help to protect the skin from the sun both from the inside and outside of the body. Damaging UVA and UVB rays may lead to skin cancer or other skin disorders besides drying and weathering the skin that exacerbates aging skin. UVA rays may penetrate deep within the thickest layer of the skin, or the dermis. UVB rays may often burn the superficial layers of the skin and may play a key role in skin cancer.

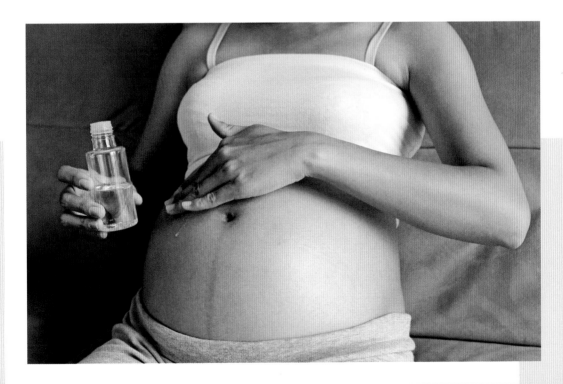

There's more than just coconut. Here are a host of other important skin care helpers.

red clover

Red clover (*Trifolium pratense*) is a commonly used remedy for treating skin conditions (such as acne, eczema, boils, and rashes). It can be applied externally, which is recorded in the traditions of Indiana, or it can be taken as a tea, which is the practice in the southern Appalachian region.

Red clover tea is also one of the most often prescribed remedies for skin conditions in professional medical herbalism in North America. Red clover was used both internally and externally for skin conditions by the Eclectic physicians at the turn of the century. Harvey Felter, a professor of medicine, said in his *King's American Dispensatory* that red clover, when applied externally, soothes inflamed skin, disinfects it, and promotes the growth of healthy tissue.

The plant contains more than thirty identified chemical constituents. Besides containing antimicrobial and anti-inflammatory chemicals, red clover also contains allantoin, which promotes the healing and growth of healthy skin tissue.

Directions: *For external use, try this remedy from Indiana: Simmer whole flowering red clover plants until tender. Use*

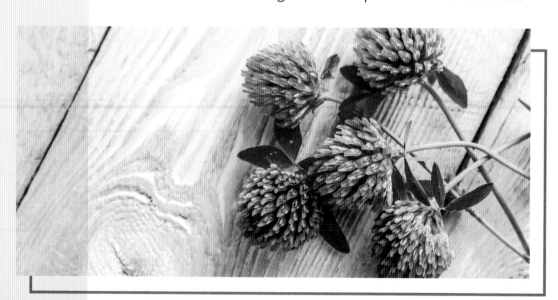

just enough water to cover. Strain, press the plants into a thick mass, and sprinkle with white flour. (The flour helps add consistency to the poultice.) Place the floured poultice directly on the irritated skin. Leave on for about half an hour. You can use the red clover poultice several times a day. (The poultice can last a few days if it's kept in the refrigerator between applications.) The poultice is designed to help reduce inflammation and promote healing.

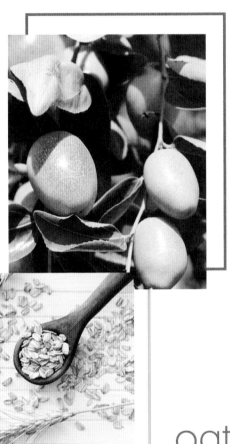

jojoba oil

The Papago Indian tribe of the Southwest has used jojoba nut (*Simmondsia chinensis*) preparations to treat skin conditions such as boils and rashes. The nuts are traditionally dried and then pulverized and applied to the skin. Jojoba oil is now commercially extracted, and it is a popular addition to skin creams, oils, and ointments available in health food stores. The oil is also used today in the traditional medicine of the Southwest for chapped skin.

Directions: *To soothe your chapped skin you can apply commercial jojoba oil as desired to skin.*

oatmeal

Oatmeal is a treatment for chapped hands in folklorist Clarence Meyer's collection of remedies called *American Folk Medicine*. In the method described below, oatmeal is used to both moisten and dry the skin.

Directions: *To treat chapped hands with oatmeal use wet oatmeal instead of soap to wash chapped hands. Then, after drying hands with a towel, rub the hands with dry oatmeal.*

clay

Clay application is a common natural remedy for treating various skin conditions throughout the world. It was common among the North American Indians even before the arrival of the European colonists. Today, the therapeutic use of clay makes up an important part of modern Seventh Day Adventist traditions. Clay is drawing and cooling. It is most effective on moist and inflamed conditions rather than on dry, chapped skin.

Directions: Purchase bentonite clay or cosmetic grade clay at a health food store or drugstore. Mix the clay with water to make a paste and apply to the skin. Allow to dry, then gently flake off after a few hours. Wipe the clay off over a bowl. Discard the waste in your garden or on your lawn, because clay can stop up your pipes. Apply clay every few hours.

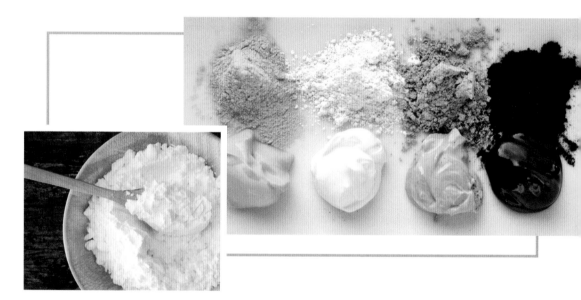

cornstarch & cornmeal

Cornstarch and cornmeal are common agents used to treat moist skin conditions such as heat rash, according to folklorist Clarence Meyer's *American Folk Medicine*. Cornstarch and cornmeal are also used to treat chapped skin and prickly heat.

Directions: You can wash the affected area, wipe it dry, and dust with cornstarch.

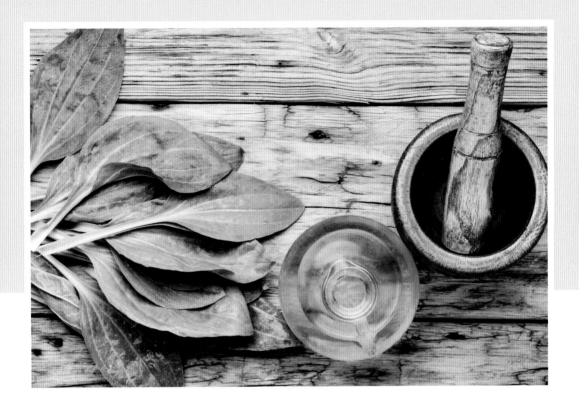

plantain leaves

Plantain leaves (*Plantago major*) are a common weed found on lawns throughout the United States. It was naturalized in North America after the arrival of the Europeans. Native Americans called it "White Man's Footprint" because it seemed to follow the European colonists wherever they went. The Delaware, Mohegan, Ojibwa, Cherokee, and other Native American tribes used plantain for treating minor wounds and insect bites.

Plantain has been used in cultures around the world to treat wounds and skin conditions. Plantain contains a pharmacy of constituents that are beneficial to the skin, including at least fifteen anti-inflammatory constituents and six analgesic chemicals. Like red clover, it contains the constituent allantoin, which promotes cell proliferation and tissue healing.

Directions: *You can crush a small handful of fresh plantain leaves and apply the juice locally to dry, chapped skin.*

Thinking About Your Skin

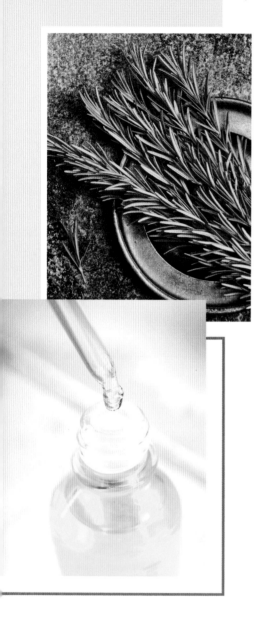

rosemary

Rosemary leaf (*Rosmarinus officinalis*) is a remedy from the Southwest for treating windburn and cracked and chapped skin. It is also used in that region (and other areas as well) as a wash for infectious skin conditions. The plant's leaf contains four anti-inflammatory substances—carnosol, oleanolic acid, rosmarinic acid, and ursolic acid. Rosemary also contains more than ten antiseptic constituents.

Directions: *To prepare you can crush rosemary leaves and warm in a pan on low heat. Add some lard to make a salve. Simmer over low heat until the lard takes on the color and aroma of the rosemary. Let cool. Apply to the affected areas as desired.*

vitamin E oil

Vitamin E oil rubbed into scar tissue will help to reduce a scar, according to the traditions of the Amish. The Amish also use cocoa butter and castor oil for the same purpose. All three oils contain vitamin E, but the vitamin E oil contains higher amounts. Vitamin E has been shown to reduce scarring in a variety of scientific experiments. Treatment with vitamin E for skin grafts after severe burns did not work in one trial, however, so there may be a limit as to what can be accomplished with this simple remedy.

Directions: *As soon as possible after a wound is closed, rub vitamin E oil into the tissues for five to ten minutes twice a day. The rubbing, which increases circulation and can break up deep scars, is an important part of the application process. Continue rubbing in the oil on a daily basis for months if necessary, or at least until improvement appears.*

Botanical Beauty

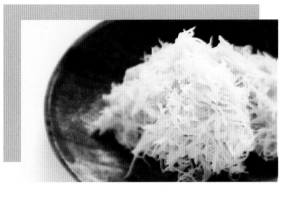

potato poultice

According to medical traditions of the Romani, a potato poultice will improve puffy skin, especially those "bags" under the eyes. This same method is taught in contemporary naturopathic medical schools to reduce inflammation of the skin.

Directions: To make a poultice, thoroughly clean two or three potatoes. Grate (including the potato skins) and press them with your hands into a paste. Apply to the affected areas of the skin. Leave in place while relaxing for fifteen minutes. Remove the poultice and clean and dry the area.

aloe vera

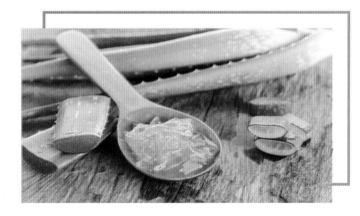

The juice of the aloe vera plant has been used as a burn remedy by practically every culture. Aloe vera is recommended as a remedy for burns, from sunburn to serious third-degree burns. Aloe vera gel also acts as a disinfectant and reduces bacteria in burns.

Directions: For a small burn, break off a leaf, slice it down the middle, and rub the gel on the skin. To make a poultice of aloe, place the cut leaf on the burned area, and wrap the area with gauze. You can also apply store-bought aloe gel or juice. An alternate formula is to extend the aloe vera sap with olive oil. Here's how: Add eight ounces of extra virgin olive oil to two ounces of fresh squeezed aloe vera sap. Apply directly to the burn area.

goldenseal

Goldenseal *(Hydrastis canadensis)* was used as a Native American remedy for skin infections, such as impetigo, even before the European colonists arrived. Its use as a topical disinfectant and internal bitter tonic spread rapidly to the English colonists in the eastern parts of the country. It has been used in one school of American medicine or another ever since. Goldenseal contains the antimicrobial substance berberine, which kills both *Streptococcus* and *Staphylococcus* bacteria, the two most common infecting agents in impetigo. Other berberine-containing plants include Oregon grape root *(Mahonia aquifolium, Berberis aquifolium)* and barberry *(Berberis vulgaris).*

Directions: *Place ½ ounce of goldenseal root bark or powder in one pint of water. Bring to a boil, then simmer for twenty minutes. Allow the water to cool to room temperature. Stir and, without straining, apply to the affected area with a clean cloth. Cover with a clean bandage or gauze pad. Reapply the application every two hours as desired.*

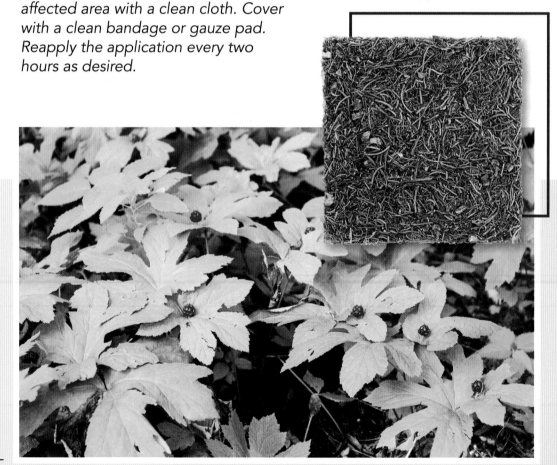

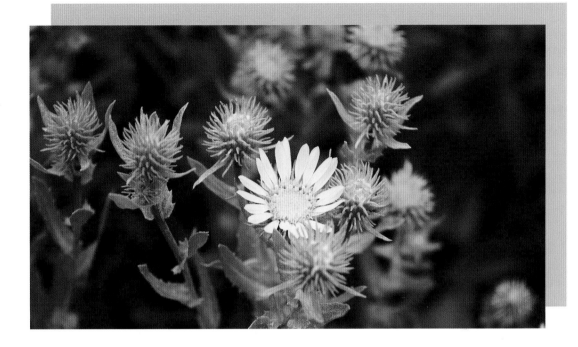

gumweed

Gumweed (*Grindelia* spp.) grows throughout the American Southwest and northwestern Mexico. It has been used as a skin remedy in those regions first by Native Americans and later by others who settled there.

Gumweed entered into the medical practice of the Eclectic physicians during the late 19th and early 20th centuries. In *The Eclectic Materia Medica, Pharmacology, and Therapeutics,* Harvey Felter states that gumweed was especially well-suited to treat those skin conditions characterized by "feeble circulation and a tendency to ulceration."

Gumweed was an official medicine in the *United States Pharmacopoeia* from 1882 until 1926. It remains an official medicine in Germany; it is used there as an expectorant for coughs. Little research has been performed into the constituents of gumweed. The resin contains anti-inflammatory constituents, so it may be useful in treating infectious or inflammatory skin conditions.

Directions: *Apply the sticky sap from the leaves or flowers of gumweed to the affected areas. Reapply every few hours. Alternately, you can purchase some tincture of gumweed and use it as a wash. Reapply the tincture every few hours.*

Thinking About Your Skin

milk

Milk can be applied to the skin to relieve the irritation and discomfort of a variety of skin ailments. The remedy is also popular in the medicine of New England. In the southern Appalachians, it is buttermilk that's preferred. These remedies traditionally used whole milk right from the cow, which, these days, is not usually available for sale.

Directions: *If you're going to try this remedy, use whole milk, not low-fat milk. The short- and medium-chain fatty acids in the butterfat of whole milk may have a mild antimicrobial effect on the skin. Any beneficial effect of this remedy is more likely due to the soothing quality of the milk rather than any actual pharmaceutical activity.*

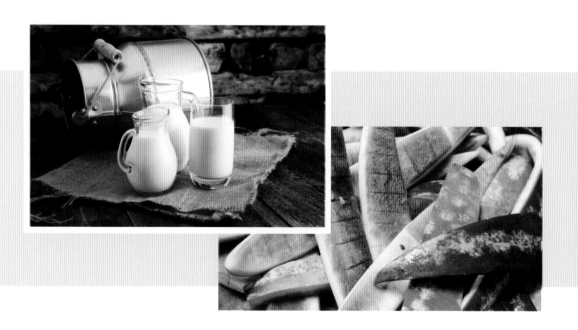

watermelon rind

To treat rash in babies, the Amish suggest rubbing the affected area with watermelon rind.

Directions: *Rub the affected area with the inside of a watermelon rind. Be sure to dry the area thoroughly and apply a talcum powder or some other drying agent.*

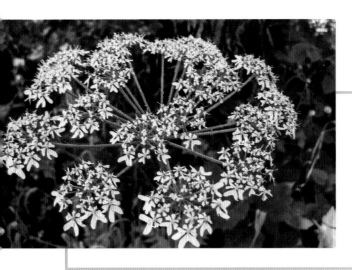

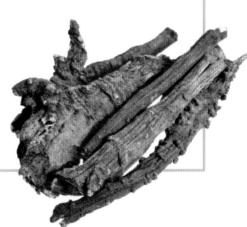

osha

Osha (*Ligusticum porteri*), which is native to the Rocky Mountains, was a panacea to the American Indians in the area. The plant remains one of the most important natural remedies of the residents of the Rio Grande Valley. Osha is used for colds, flu, bronchitis, and also as a skin wash for superficial infections.

Very little scientific research has been performed into either the constituents or the pharmaceutical properties of the plant, but a close Chinese relative of the plant (*Ligusticum wallichi*) has been studied extensively. The main constituent of its aromatic oil is alpha-pinene, which has antimicrobial and disinfectant properties. Constituents called ligustilides have broad spectrum antibiotic effects as well as antiviral and antifungal properties.

Directions: *Using a coffee grinder, grind a piece of osha root into a powder. Spread the powder in a small skillet. Add enough lard or butter to cover the powder when melted. Put on low heat until the lard or butter is melted. Stir well and let stand at room temperature until the salve becomes solid. To treat a skin infection, apply the salve to the skin every two to three hours.*

Alternately, mix the osha with enough honey to make a paste. Apply to a piece of gauze and use a bandage to hold in place over the affected area. Osha may irritate the skin. If this occurs, reduce the frequency of the treatments or try another remedy.

Thinking About Your Skin

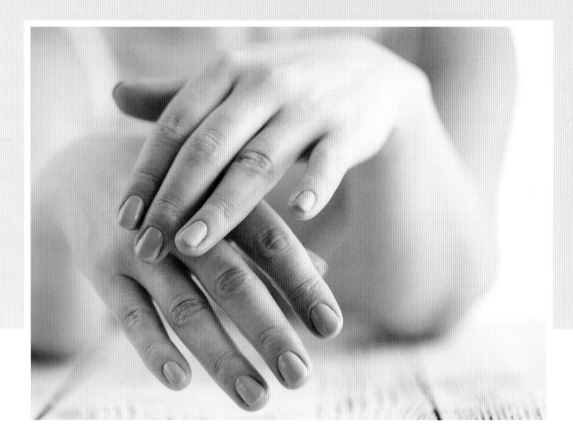

urine

Urine therapy for cleansing wounds and treating skin infections appeared in the ancient medical systems. Urine contains the substance urea, a disinfectant and skin moistener used in modern pharmaceutical preparations to cleanse wounds and in cosmetic products. (It is animal urine that is used in these preparations, of course.)

Directions: *Apply fresh warm urine to chapped hands and skin and allow skin to air dry.*

salves & ointments

Homemade salves and ointments are commonly used throughout the world. To make one, a medicinal plant is cooked or mixed in lard, butter, beeswax, or other oily substance that remains solid at room temperature. The oily portion of the salve helps to soften and penetrate the tissues and also serves to hold the medicinal portion in place.

To make a simple salve, chop, powder, crush, or grind the medicinal material as small as possible and place in the bottom of a skillet or a slow cooker. Place enough lard, butter, or beeswax in the pan or pot; it should cover the plant material when melted. Leave on very lowest heat for a while—at least ten to twenty minutes for a leafy substance, forty to sixty minutes for roots. Remove from heat. Let the ointment cool to a solid state. Store lard or butter ointments in the refrigerator. Plantain, grindelia, goldenseal, rosemary, and osha are all easy to make into salves. Combinations of the herbs may make more effective salves than single herb preparations.

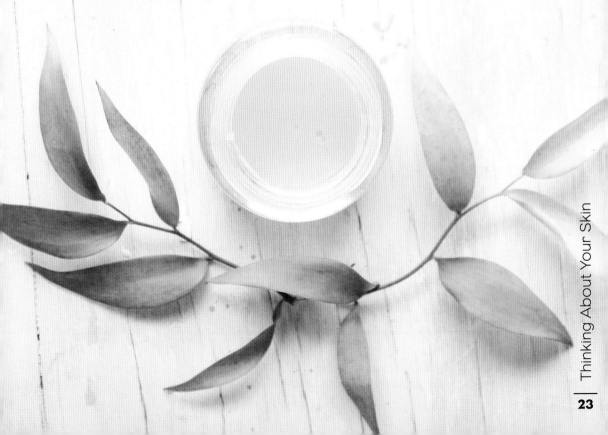

Chapter 2

TACKLING COMMON SKIN CONDITIONS

Now that we know more about coconut and other common skin care remedies, let's investigate common skin conditions and how to tackle them.

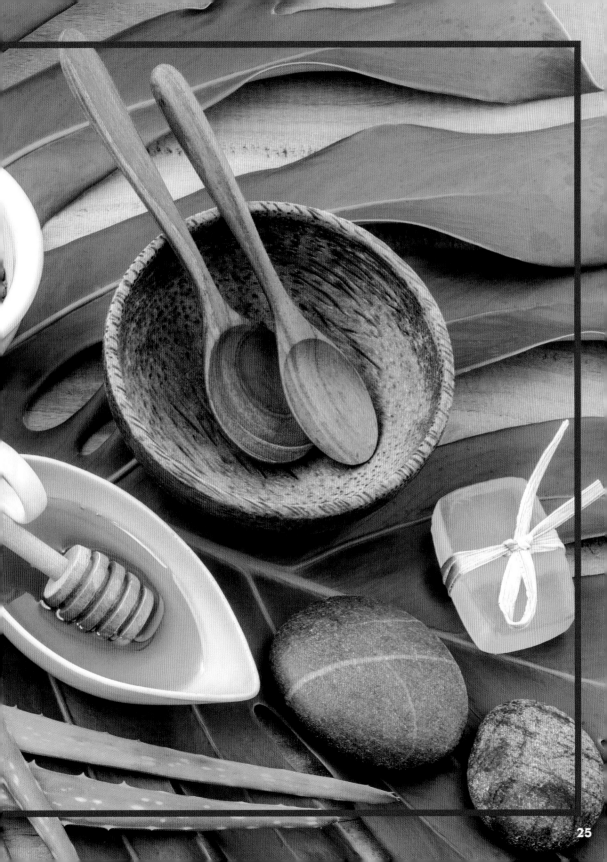

Burns & Sunburns

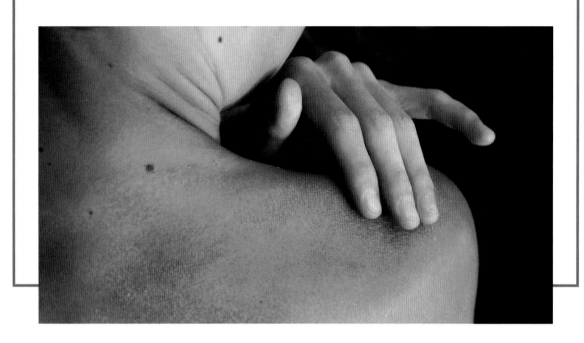

Burns are medically classified in two ways: by the depth of the burn and by the amount of body area the burn covers. Deep burns and burns covering large surface areas require medical examination.

The most superficial burn is the first-degree burn, which is typical of a simple sunburn. A second-degree burn penetrates deeper into the skin and is usually accompanied by blisters. Third-degree burns involve deep tissue destruction. Third-degree burns may not blister, so they at first may appear to be less serious than they are. Often the skin looks whitish or charred. The chief risk of second- and third-degree burns is infection, and the more surface area that is affected, the more serious the risk. Infection may enter through ruptured blisters or through seemingly intact skin that has been burned.

Many remedies are inappropriate for these burns, and some could actually promote infection. Conventional treatment for simple superficial burns includes cooling the tissues as soon as possible to reduce inflammation and blistering, and applying soothing ointments.

remedies for burns & sunburns

Vinegar

Vinegar is both astringent and antiseptic, and like cool water, it helps to prevent blisters.

Directions: You can apply vinegar to the burn every few minutes. Dilute the vinegar if the skin is very sensitive.

Honey

Honey is a universal natural remedy to disinfect wounds and burns throughout the world. Honey naturally attracts water, and, when applied to a burn or wound, draws fluids out of the tissues, cleaning the wound.

Furthermore, most bacteria cannot live in the presence of honey. Honey is sometimes applied to gauze and used to dress severe burns in conventional medicine.

Directions: You can apply honey to a piece of sterile gauze, and place directly on the burn, honey side to the skin. Change the dressing three to four times a day. Be sure to seek medical attention for serious burns.

emergency burn wash/compress

-5 drops lavender oil
-1 pint water, about 50 degrees Fahrenheit

Directions: Add the essential oil to the water and stir well to disperse the oil. Immerse the burned area for several minutes, or take a soft cloth, soak it in the water, and apply it to the burn. Leave the compress on for several minutes, then soak again and reapply at least twice more.

sunburn soother

-20 drops lavender oil
-4 ounces aloe vera juice
-200 IU vitamin E oil
-1 tablespoon vinegar

Directions: Combine ingredients. Shake well before using. Keep this remedy in a spritzer bottle, and use it as often as needed. If you keep the spray in the refrigerator, the coolness will provide extra relief. For the best healing, make sure you use aloe vera juice and not drugstore gel.

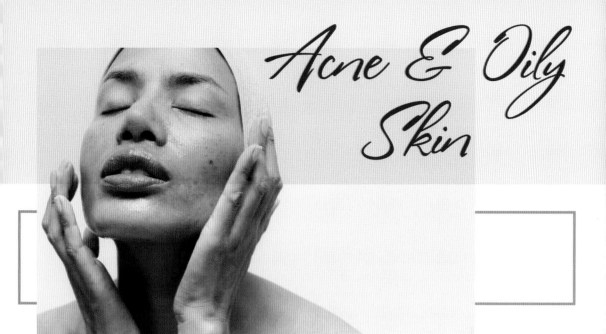

Acne & Oily Skin

Acne often begins with the normal hormonal changes of puberty. The hormone testosterone increases at that time in both men and women and causes an increase in the size and secretions of the sebaceous glands in the skin that produce sebum (an oily secretion). Most excess oil produced by these glands leaves the skin through the hair follicles (the tubelike structures from which hairs develop). Sometimes, however, oil clogs these tubes and creates comedones (blocked hair follicles).

If comedones are open to the surface of the skin, they are called blackheads. They contain sebum from the sebaceous glands, bacteria, and any skin tissue that accumulates near the surface. Comedones that are closed at the surface are called whiteheads.

Clogged hair follicles can rupture internally, resulting in a discharge of their contents into the surrounding tissues. Bacteria in the injured area can sometimes lead to more widespread inflammation and the formation of painful cysts. In severe cases, pitting and scarring result.

Acne normally resolves all by itself without specific medical treatment. For some individuals, however, acne can continue into the adult years. In women, acne may cycle with the menses, due to varying output of hormones. Oily cosmetics or moisturizers can sometimes cause acne or make an existing case worse. And although a link has not been medically proven, many people notice acne flare-ups when they're under stress.

Tackling Common Skin Conditions

Acne has no prevention or cure, but there are several treatments. The main treatment for mild acne is thorough cleansing with a mild soap two to three times a day. Some over-the-counter medications, particularly lotions or creams containing benzoyl peroxide, can help troubled skin as well. For persistent acne, a doctor might prescribe an antibiotic preparation that can be applied to the surface of the skin or an oral antibiotic, such as tetracycline. Antibiotics do not heal the pimples or prevent their formation, but they do prevent their infection or rupture, and subsequent inflammation of the surrounding tissues. Thus, antibiotics may also help to prevent scarring. Unfortunately, oral antibiotics can also kill the friendly bacteria in the intestinal tract and cause unpleasant digestive side effects, such as gas, bloating, and indigestion. Antibiotics may also promote intestinal or vaginal yeast infections.

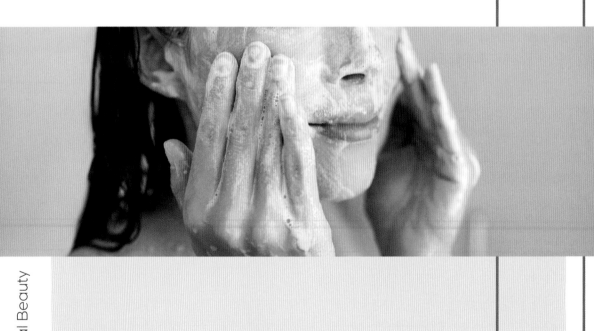

remedies for acne & oily skin

Clay Packs

Many remedies call for
the use of astringent
washes and poultices.
These remedies naturally
absorb or "draw" the
excess oily secretions
out of the skin.

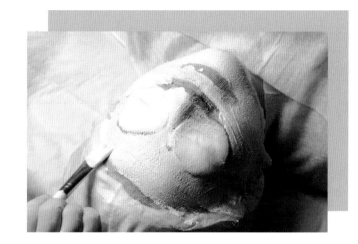

*Directions: Applying
clay packs to the face is
a popular acne remedy.
You can purchase cosmetic grade clay for the same purpose.*

Burdock

Burdock tea has been used to treat acne throughout the eastern states and
at least as far west as Indiana. Burdock *(Arctium lappa)* is slightly diaphoretic,
which means it brings blood circulation to the surface of the skin to promote
sweating. The increased local circulation of immune elements of the blood
may help fight the infection and inflammation of acne.

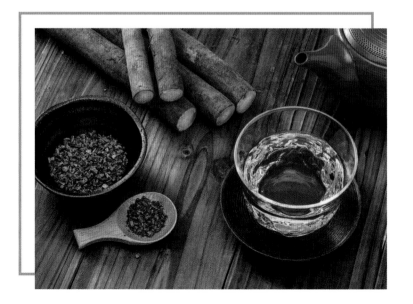

*Directions:
Burdock contains
a high amount of
starch, and, applied
locally, the starch
may help absorb
excess oils from
the skin.*

toner for oily complexions

-12 drops lemongrass oil

-6 drops juniper berry oil

-2 drops ylang ylang oil

-1 ounce witch hazel lotion

-1 ounce aloe vera gel

Directions: Combine all of the ingredients in a glass bottle. Give the mixture a good shake and it's done! Apply at least once a day. If you find witch hazel too drying, vinegar is an excellent substitute. It is not as drying as the witch hazel lotion and helps to retain the skin's natural acid balance.

zit zap compress

-4 drops cedarwood oil

-2 drops eucalyptus oil

-1 teaspoon Epsom salts

-1/4 cup water

Directions: Pour the boiling water over the Epsom salts. When the salts are dissolved and the water has cooled just enough to not burn the skin, add the essential oils. Soak a small absorbent cloth in the hot solution, then press the cloth against the blemishes for about one minute. Repeat several times by rewetting the cloth in the same solution.

Itches & Rashes

An itch may be due to local irritation of the skin. Local irritation may be caused by insect bites, stings, or infestation; by an allergic reaction to a plant, animal, or synthetic substance; or by infection from molds, yeasts, or other microorganisms. Sometimes itching can be simply due to dry skin. Many prescription drugs can also cause itching.

An itch may also be due to a systemic disease—one that's irritating the skin from the inside out. For example, disorders of the blood, kidneys, or thyroid can cause itching. An itch from a systemic disease may affect only a small area of the skin, as in cases of eczema or psoriasis or allergies to substances that have been eaten. Sometimes a systemic disease will cause itching over large areas of the body or itching that moves from one place to another.

Conventional treatment of itching and rashes first requires an investigation of the cause of the skin condition. For example, if itching is the result of an allergic sensitivity to a certain fabric, avoiding that particular fabric is likely to be recommended. If prescription drugs are responsible for your discomfort, your physician may prescribe a different medication.

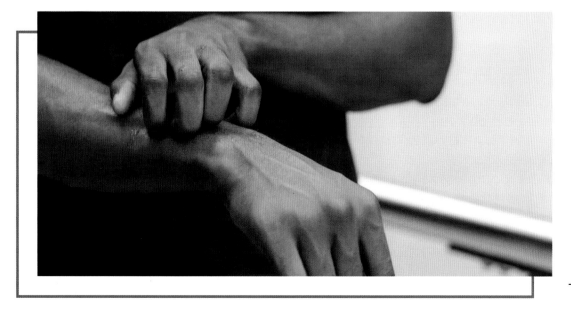

remedies for itches & rashes

Juniper-Clove Salve

Folklorist Clarence Meyer's *American Folk Medicine* suggests using a salve of juniper *(Juniperus* spp.) and clove *(Eugenia carophyllata)* to soothe itchy skin. Juniper contains anti-inflammatory volatile substances, and clove contains the substance eugenol, a topical anesthetic widely used by dentists. The eugenol presumably affects the itch by numbing the nerve endings in the skin.

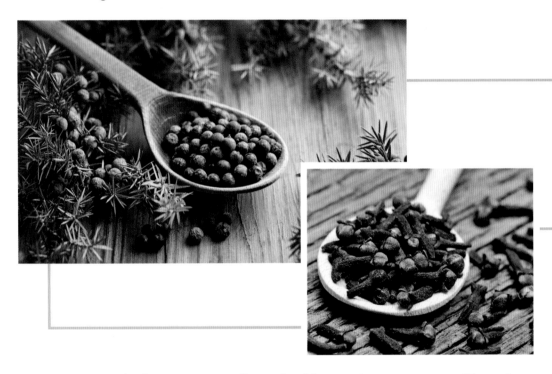

Directions: Melt three ounces of unsalted butter in a saucepan. Then, in a separate pan, melt a lump of beeswax about the size of two tablespoons (it is difficult to get beeswax actually into the tablespoon). When the beeswax is melted, add it to the melted butter and stir well. Add five tablespoons of ground juniper berries and three tablespoons of ground clove to the butter/beeswax mixture and stir. (Instead of purchasing herbs as powders, it is best to grind the herbs yourself because the volatile substances are preserved better in the whole berries and clove.) Allow the mixture to cool and become solid. Apply as a salve to itchy skin.

Lemon Juice

The aromatic substances in lemon have anesthetic and anti-inflammatory properties, which may be responsible for its medicinal activity, if any in fact exists.

Directions: *Juice a lemon. Apply undiluted to itchy skin as needed until condition improves.*

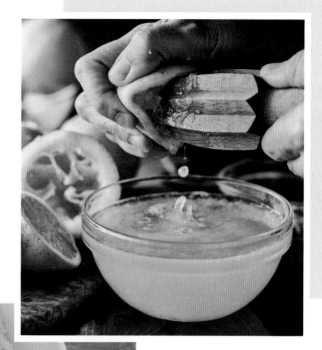

Mung Bean Paste

A treatment for heat rash or prickly is mung bean "soap," which is made from a mixture of cooked mung beans and sugar. The most important component of the formula may be the sugar, however, because by nature it is drying and cooling. Sugar has been used in various cultures to cleanse wounds. The astringent and drying properties of the beans may also have a beneficial effect on the rash.

Directions: *Cook mung beans until they can be mashed into the consistency of a paste. Add enough sugar so that the beans are sweet to the taste. Apply to the affected area, rubbing as if the paste were soap. Leave the paste in place for ten to fifteen minutes. Then remove, dry the area well, and dust with talcum powder or another drying agent.*

Eczema is an inflammation of the skin and is most commonly equated with the medical term atopic dermatitis. It is characterized by red, oozing, and sometimes crusty lesions on the face, the scalp, the extremities, and the diaper area in infants. The lesions may also become infected with bacteria or other microorganisms, and infection with herpes virus can cause serious illness. Stress, food allergens, scratching, bathing, and sweating may also induce attacks.

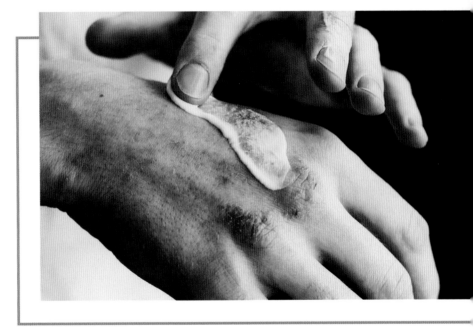

Conventional treatment includes avoidance of triggers and administration of antihistamine topical steroid creams and antibiotics for infections of the eczema lesions. Alternative medical treatments include avoidance of triggers; optimizing vitamin, mineral, and essential fatty acid nutrition to reduce tendency to develop inflammation; internal or topical applications of anti-inflammatory or soothing herbs; and administration of bitter herbs to "stimulate the liver" and optimize digestion.

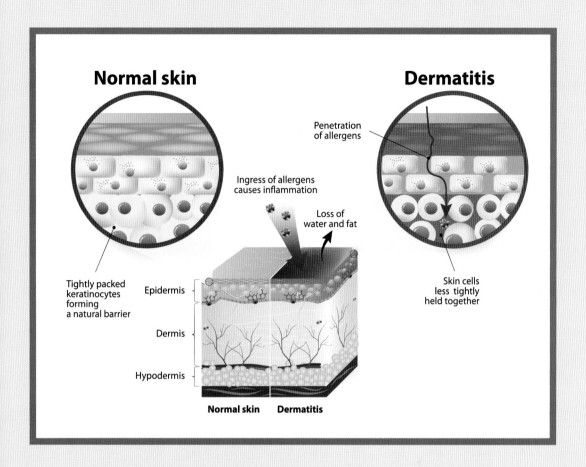

Normal skin

Dermatitis

Penetration
of allergens

Ingress of allergens
causes inflammation

Loss of
water and fat

Tightly packed
keratinocytes
forming
a natural barrier

Skin cells
less tightly
held together

Epidermis

Dermis

Hypodermis

Normal skin   **Dermatitis**

In alternative medicine, it is believed that to heal the skin, you must heal the digestive tract as well. Thus, a three-way link that exists between the liver, the digestive tract, and the skin is a key tenet of alternative medicine for treating allergic eczema and other skin inflammation. One physiological basis for this theory may be the detoxifying role of the liver. The liver normally transforms toxic substances so they can be excreted from the body either in the form of bile from the liver or as urine. If the liver is not doing its job, toxic substances may circulate freely in the body and irritate the skin "from the inside out."

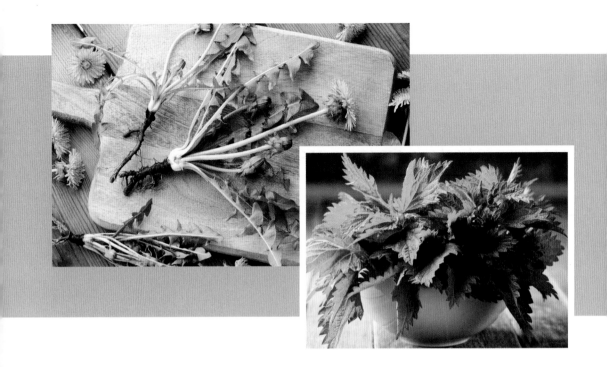

remedies for eczema & dermatitis

Nettle & Dandelion

A Romani remedy for eczema uses a combination of two "blood purifying" herbs that are traditionally prescribed to treat skin conditions. Stinging nettle *(Urtica dioica, U. urens)* has been used as an aid for healing skin conditions.

Dandelion root is traditionally considered to be a "liver" herb—its use in this country is consistent with the traditional idea of treating skin ailments through the liver. Dandelion contains both antioxidant and anti-inflammatory constituents.

Directions: *Place one ounce of dandelion root and one ounce of nettle leaf in a pot, and cover with three pints of water. Boil and then simmer, covered, on low heat for forty minutes. Cool to room temperature. Drink three cups a day. Do this for three weeks, and then take a break for seven to ten days before starting again.*

Burdock Root

In the traditional herbalism of Europe and North America, burdock (*Arctium lappa, A. minus*) is probably the most well-known for treating skin complaints such as acne, boils, or eczema. It has been used to treat skin conditions, and it is used today in natural medicine as a "blood purifier." Burdock was an official medicine in the *United States Pharmacopoeia* from 1831 until 1842, and again from 1851 until 1916; it was prescribed as a diuretic, mild laxative, and treatment for skin ailments.

Modern scientific studies show that constituents in burdock root have anti-inflammatory properties. Its constituent polysaccharide inulin, which can make up fifty percent of the root by weight, provides food for the "friendly" strains of bacteria in the gut and may thus help reduce the toxic load on the liver and skin by reducing toxicity in the bowels.

For some individuals, however, burdock can worsen eczema. Perhaps this is because burdock promotes light sweating, and sweat can trigger eczema in some people. If you find that burdock makes your eczema worse, stop using it immediately and try a different remedy.

Directions: Put one ounce of burdock root in one quart of water. Bring to a boil and simmer, covered, for forty minutes. Drink the quart throughout the day. Burdock is a mild herb and can be consumed this way for long periods of time.

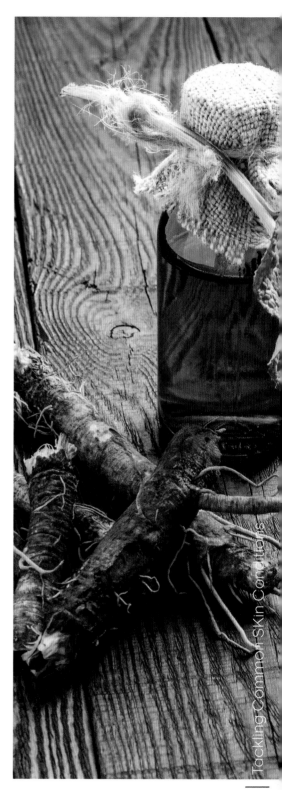

Tackling Common Skin Conditions

Yellow Dock

Yellow dock (*Rumex crispus*), like dandelion and burdock, is a traditional bitter, liver-stimulating herb. It was a remedy for treating eczema of residents of the eastern states in the 1800s. It was listed in the *United States Pharmacopoeia* from 1860 until 1890; physicians used it to treat chronic skin ailments.

Directions: *Make a tincture of yellow dock by placing four ounces of the dried root in a one-quart jar and filling the jar with 100 proof vodka or gin. Let stand for three weeks, shaking the jar once a day. Strain and store in a cool dark place. The dose is two to three droppers twice a day, taken in a cup of warm water. Alternately, you can purchase a tincture of yellow dock at a health food or herb store.*

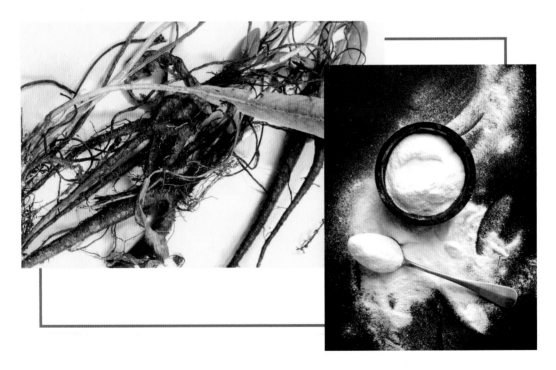

Baking Soda Bath

Contemporary Seventh Day Adventists recommend treating eczema by taking a baking soda bath. The same treatment is also used for relieving hives, itching, rashes, and other skin conditions.

Directions: *Place a few handfuls of baking soda in warm bath water and take a long soak.*

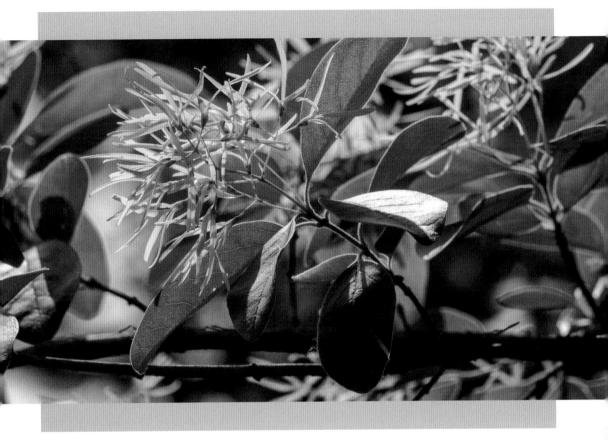

Fringe Tree Bark

A contemporary Appalachian treatment for eczema is taking fringe tree bark (*Chionanthus virginicus*). This bitter, liver-stimulating herb was one of the top ten most-often prescribed herbs by the Eclectic physicians in 1920; they used it to treat liver diseases in particular.

Though fringe tree bark has been studied very little by modern scientists, its reputation persists thanks to its former popularity. Internal use requires a tincture. Use as a tea when applying as an external wash.

Directions: *Purchase a tincture of fringe tree bark at a health food store. Take a dropperful three times a day for seven to ten days. Discontinue if any digestive discomfort develops.*

To apply as an external wash, simmer one tablespoon of the bark in a cup of boiling water for fifteen minutes. Strain and, using gauze, apply to the eczema.

Oregon Grape Root & Yellow Dock

Native American tribes took Oregon grape internally to treat the digestive tract and applied it externally to treat skin conditions. The Cowlitz tribe applied it externally as a disinfectant; today, physicians in Germany use it in the same way for treating psoriasis.

The contemporary Amish use a combination of Oregon grape root (*Berberis aquifolium*) and yellow dock root (*Rumex crispus*) for treating eczema. Oregon grape, like yellow dock, is considered in contemporary British and North American herbalism to be a liver herb, and its constituents berberine, berbamine, and oxyacanthine all promote the flow of bile.

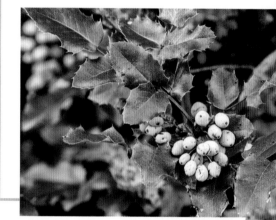

Directions: Purchase a tincture of Oregon grape root and some capsules of powdered yellow dock root. Take one dropper of the Oregon grape tincture and four capsules of the yellow dock root three times a day until the eczema is relieved. In addition, dilute one ounce of the Oregon grape tincture with five ounces of water, and apply the diluted solution, using gauze or a clean cloth, to the eczema.

Thyme

Another traditional remedy for treating eczema is to wash the affected area with a tea of thyme leaves (*Thymus vulgaris*). Thyme leaves contain about two percent thymol, a volatile constituent that has strong antiseptic and anti-inflammatory properties.

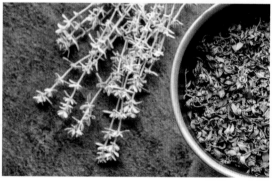

Directions: Place one ounce of thyme leaves in a one-quart canning jar and fill with boiling water. Cover tightly to prevent the thymol from escaping with the steam. Let cool to room temperature. Apply to eczema with gauze or a clean cloth three or four times a day. If you find the remedy irritating, dilute it in half and try again.

dermatitis skin care

-8 drops tea tree oil

-8 drops chamomile oil

-1 teaspoon Oregon grape tincture

-2 ounces healing salve

Directions: With a toothpick, stir the tincture and essential oils into the salve. This will make the salve semi-liquid. You can purchase the tincture at a natural food store. Apply one to four times a day.

dry complexion scrub

-6 drops lavender oil

-2 drops peppermint oil

-1 tablespoon dried elder flowers, lavender, or chamomile (optional)

-2 tablespoons oatmeal

-1 tablespoon cornmeal

Directions: Grind dry ingredients in a blender or electric coffee grinder. (Drug stores sell colloidal oatmeal, which needs no grinding.) Add the essential oils, and stir to distribute. Store in a closed container, and use instead of soap for cleansing your face. For clean skin, moisten 1 teaspoon with enough water to make a paste, dampen your face with a little water, then gently apply scrub. Rinse with warm water. Use this daily instead of soap.

Bites & Stings

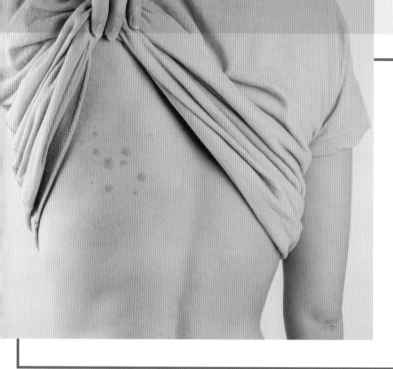

When bees, wasps, scorpions, and snakes attack humans, it's usually because we threatened them or their living space. On the other hand, insects such as mosquitoes, biting flies, ticks, chiggers, and fleas are predatory pests that view humans as good opportunities for a bite to eat. Their bites are more likely to be itchy than painful. With any bite or sting, the species' venom, or sometimes the tiny insect itself penetrates the barriers of the body. The combination of the effects of the poison and the body's attempt to eliminate it can cause pain, swelling, or itching near the bite site.

Most bites and stings are not a serious medical concern, but there are a few exceptions. In some people, the stings of bees, wasps, and hornets can cause a potentially fatal allergic reaction called anaphylactic shock. Any shortness of breath, difficulty breathing, or swelling in the airway after a sting is a medical emergency requiring immediate attention. Tick bites can cause Lyme disease or Rocky Mountain spotted fever. Bites of the black widow spider and brown recluse spider can cause serious medical symptoms; any reaction following a spider bite requires medical attention.

The bites of the poisonous snakes in North America are not usually life threatening to healthy adults. Of about eight thousand such bites in the United States each year, fewer than fifteen cause fatalities; the deaths occur mostly in children and the elderly. The illness from a poisonous snake bite can be quite severe, however, and should be treated as a medical emergency. Any snake bite can cause an infected puncture wound, which requires careful cleaning and medical attention.

The *Centruroides exilicauda* scorpion, native to Arizona, New Mexico, and the California side of the Colorado River, is the only North American scorpion that can cause serious illness or death. The folk remedies here are for normal itches and pains associated with bites and stings, not for the more exotic complications caused by Lyme disease, anaphylactic shock, or snake bites.

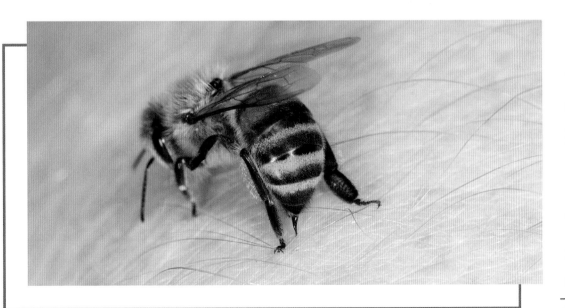

remedies for bites & stings

Mints

Native American tribes have used various species of mint for the relief and prevention of insect bites. For example, peppermint *(Mentha piperita)* contains camphor, which is cooling to the skin and helps relieve itching.

Directions: Place one ounce of peppermint leaf in a one-quart canning jar and cover with boiling water. Seal the jar and let stand until the water cools to room temperature.

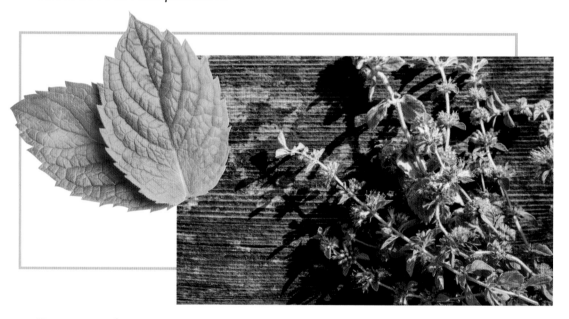

Pennyroyal

Early American colonists introduced European pennyroyal to North America, but found that Native Americans were already using American pennyroyal *(Hedeoma pulegioides)*. The herb was used for centuries to prevent deer tick bites. In the Frank C. Brown *Collection of North Carolina Folklore*, a North Carolina source says: "Pennyroyal beaten on the legs will keep insects away." Pennyroyal contains eleven separate constituents with identified insect-repellent properties."

Directions: Purchase the essential oil of pennyroyal. Put eight to ten drops in some almond oil, mix, and apply—especially around the ankles, neck, and scalp—to repel ticks and other insects.

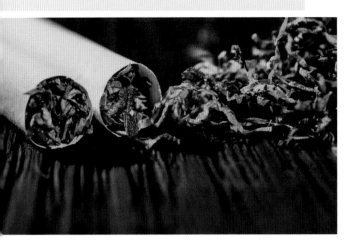

Tobacco

Some Native American tribes moistened the leaves of wild tobacco (*Nicotiana rustica, N. glauca*) with saliva and applied the leaves to a bite or sting. The Six Nations, a league of Indians that extended from the Hudson River to Lake Erie, also used tobacco to treat insect bites. Using tobacco in this manner later passed into Appalachian folk medicine, where tobacco poultices are still used today to treat bee, hornet, yellow jacket, and wasp stings as well as spider bites. In the folk medicine of the Southwest, a strong tobacco tea is applied to tick bites to help draw the tick out.

Directions: Mix tobacco from cigarettes, cigars, chewing tobacco, or snuff with water and apply directly to a bite or sting.

Plantain Leaves

Plantain (*Plantago* spp.) is the common four-leafed weed that grows in lawns and around sidewalks throughout the country. The plant has been adopted as a medicine for treating bites, stings, and minor wounds. Plantain's chemical constituents may explain its ability to soothe pain and promote wound healing.

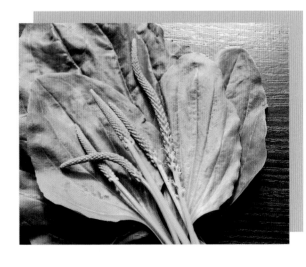

Directions: Crush a small handful of fresh plantain leaves and apply locally to bites and stings. Applied externally, the plant stimulates and cleanses the skin and encourages wounds to heal faster. You can apply fresh leaves every fifteen to twenty minutes. Leave on as long as desired.

Tackling Common Skin Conditions

Vinegar

Folklore recommends a vinegar wash for treating bites and stings.

Directions: Use undiluted vinegar as a wash to stop itching or to relieve the pain of stings. Also, you can try this Romani recipe: Take a handful of thyme (Thymus vulgaris) *and seal it in a bottle of vinegar for one cycle of the moon, in the sun if possible. Shake the bottle every morning and evening. Then, after an additional half cycle of the moon, crush seven garlic cloves and add them to the bottle. At the end of the second lunar cycle, strain and bottle the liquid. Use as a wash for itchy or infected bites.*

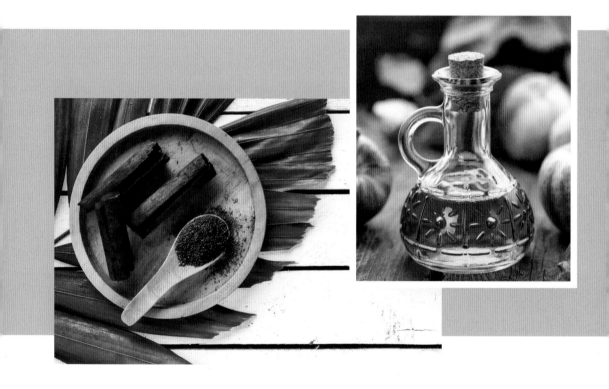

Charcoal

A charcoal poultice treats insect and snake bites. Charcoal has strong drawing properties and is sometimes taken internally to neutralize ingested poisons in the gut.

Directions: Use as much crushed charcoal as you need to cover the injured area. Place the charcoal directly over the area and cover with a clean cloth. Replace the poultice every ten to fifteen minutes until relief is obtained.

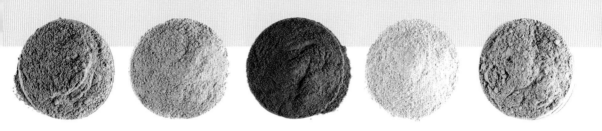

Clay

Using clay or mud packs to treat bee and wasp stings is a universal folk remedy. Some people believe it works by literally drawing the toxins out.

Directions: Apply mud or cold clay (any kind of clay soil or cosmetic clay will do) to the sting area to relieve pain and reduce swelling. When the clay dries, apply new clay. Repeat this as long as necessary.

essential oils

For mosquito or other insect bites that don't demand much attention, a simple dab of essential oil of lavender or tea tree provides relief from itching. Chamomile and lavender essential oils reduce swelling and inflammation, and diminish itching or other allergic responses. Bentonite clay poultices are of great help for more painful stings or bites. As the clay dries, it pulls toxins to the skin's surface to keep them from spreading, and it pulls out pus or stingers embedded in the skin. Adding essential oil to clay keeps the clay reconstituted, preserved, and ready for an emergency. If an allergic reaction, such as excessive itching, swelling and inflammation, or difficulty breathing, occurs following a bite, call a doctor immediately.

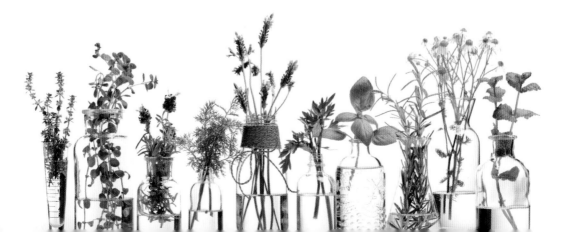

bug-off repellent

-12 drops citronella oil
-12 drops eucalyptus oil
-6 drops cedarwood oil
-6 drops geranium oil
-1 ounce rubbing alcohol or vodka

Directions: *Mix ingredients together, and dab on exposed skin. This recipe contains a lot of essential oil and is highly concentrated, so don't use it like a massage oil. Rubbing alcohol is poisonous if drunk, so if you use it, be sure to mark the container accordingly. Pat on as needed. Since it won't harm fabrics (except silk), use some of it on your clothes so that you won't apply too much to your skin or absorb too much through the skin.*

bite and sting poultice

-12 drops lavender oil
-5 drops chamomile oil
-1 tablespoon bentonite clay
-2 teaspoons distilled water

Directions: *Put clay in the container to be stored. Add the water slowly, stirring more in as the clay absorbs them. Add essential oils, stirring to distribute them evenly. The resulting mixture should be a thick paste. If necessary, add more distilled water to achieve this consistency. Store the paste in a container with a tight lid to slow dehydration. It should last several months, but if the mixture starts to dry out, add a little distilled water to reconstitute it. Use as much and as often as needed.*

Simple cuts and scrapes can easily be treated with antiseptic essential oils. A mist of diluted oil is an excellent way to apply them. Herbal salves containing antiseptic essential oils are also effective in treating scrapes or wounds that aren't too deep. Need to protect your cut? Many of the resins and balsams such as benzoin, frankincense, and myrrh actually form a protective barrier over the wound that acts as an antiseptic "Band-Aid." In an emergency, don't forget that you can dab a little lavender or tea tree oil directly on a scrape as they are among the least irritating of oils.

Essential oils for cuts and scrapes include: benzoin, eucalyptus, frankincense, geranium, lavender, lemon, myrrh, rose, and tea tree.

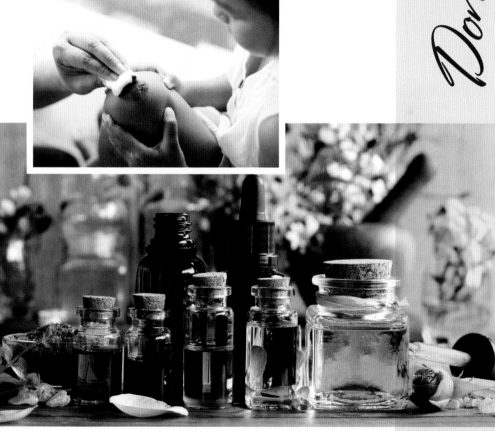

Hives are rashlike, itchy skin bumps that are most often seen in children, but anyone can get them. They are often caused by a food allergy, although it may be difficult to diagnose at first because the reaction can occur hours or even a day after eating the culprit food. While it's a good idea to eliminate the allergen and build up the immune system, the immediate need is to stop the itching.

The essential oil of chamomile is an excellent first choice to treat hives, but if it's too expensive or you don't have any on hand, you can turn to an essential oil that decreases inflammation, such as lavender. The fragrance of either lavender or chamomile oil can also be very calming to someone who feels that they are going to go mad from the itching.

First wash off the skin. If the itching is not sufficiently relieved, apply the Hives Paste. A child who normally objects to having a poultice smeared on his or her skin will often accept this poultice because it so effectively stops the itching.

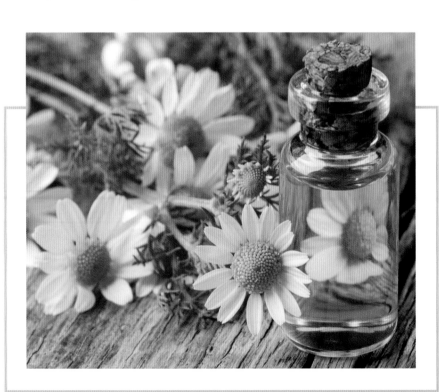

hives skin wash

-5 drops chamomile or 10 drops lavender oil

-2 drops peppermint oil

-3 tablespoons baking soda

-2 cups water (or use peppermint tea instead)

Directions: Combine the ingredients. If you are making a tea to use as the base instead of water, pour 2 ½ cups of boiling water over 4 teaspoons of dried peppermint leaves, and steep 15 minutes. Strain out the herb. Add the remaining ingredients. Use a soft cloth or a skin sponge to apply on irritated skin until itching is alleviated. Chamomile is the best choice for this recipe, but it is expensive, so 10 drops of lavender essential oil can be substituted, if necessary.

hives paste

-1/4 cup of the Hives Skin Wash

-3 tablespoons bentonite clay

Directions: Stir the ingredients into a paste, and wait about five minutes for it to thicken. Apply to irritated skin with your fingers or a wooden tongue depressor. Let dry on skin, and leave for at least 45 minutes before washing off. Reapply for another 30 minutes if the area is still itching.

Chapter 3

FIGHTING COLDS, FEVERS, AND INFLUENZA

At some point in our lives, a nasty cold, fever, or influenza is likely to knock the wind out of our sails. The herbs and remedies found in this chapter are beneficial when dealing with the effects of these unpleasant illnesses.

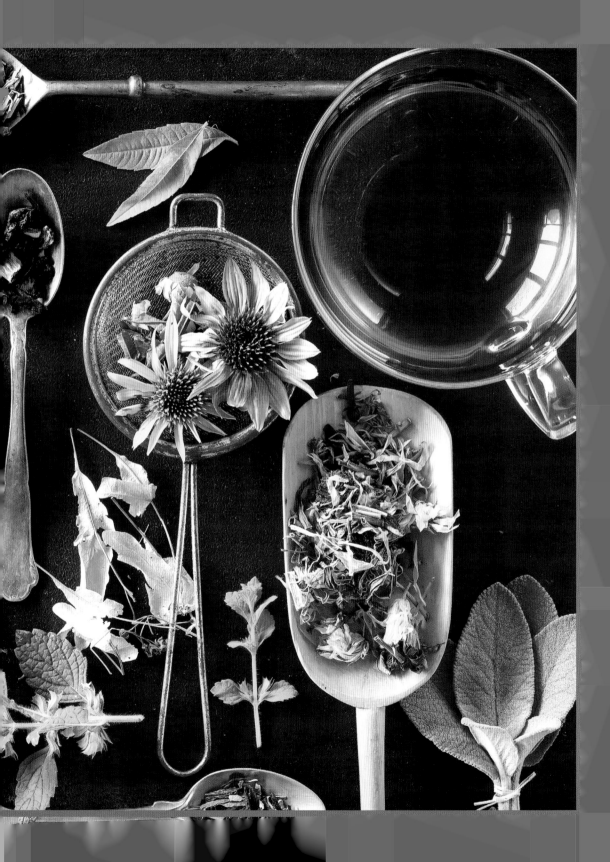

Although we often say "colds and flu" in the same breath, influenza is a very different disease from the common cold.

The influenza virus takes up residence mainly in the throat and bronchial tract. If you have the flu, you usually have a fever, and a fever is not usually present in a cold. The fever usually passes within three days, but the fatigue, muscle aches, and cough that result from the flu can linger for weeks. Influenza will not seriously injure a normally healthy person, but those with preexisting lung conditions, the elderly, and others with weakened resistance are especially prone to the flu's deadly effects.

Even more serious than influenza is the novel coronavirus, SARS-CoV-2. COVID-19, the disease caused by the virus, shares overlapping symptoms with influenza. The disease attacks both the upper and lower respiratory systems, which can result in serious lung damage, pneumonia, organ failure, and even death.

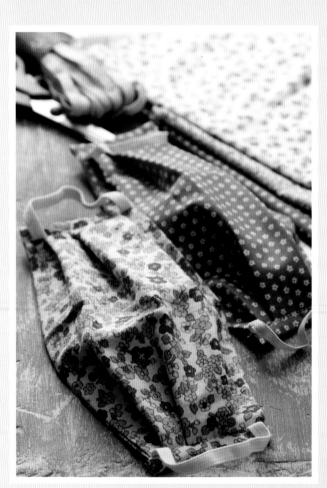

COVID-19 is much deadlier than influenza. Therapeutics and vaccines are in development to treat the disease. In the interim, public health officials say social distancing measures, as well as the use of face masks in public, are essential to curtailing the spread of the novel coronavirus.

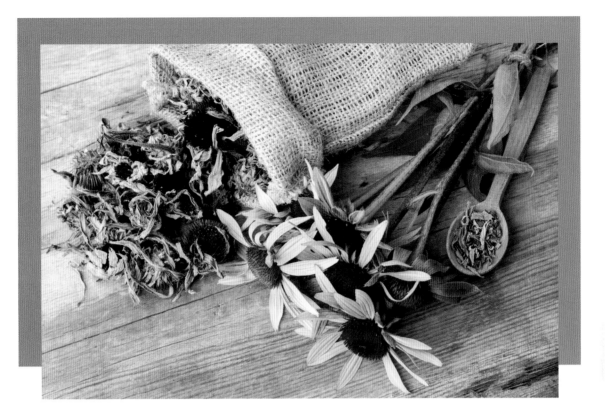

Echinacea

Echinacea (*Echinacea angustifolia, Echinacea purpurea)* is, without a doubt, the most commonly used natural remedy for treating colds and flu in the United States today. In fact, echinacea is the best-selling medicinal herb in the country.

Eclectic physicians, a now-defunct North American school of doctors who used herbs as medicines, adopted the use of echinacea in the mid-1880s. By 1920, it was the remedy they prescribed the most. The use of echinacea spread to Germany in the 1930s, where it remains an approved medicine today—used to treat colds, flu, and other conditions related to underlying deficiencies of the immune system.

Directions: Echinacea is famous in contemporary medical herbalism for its ability to "abort" a cold or flu. German clinical trials show that echinacea, taken preventively during cold and flu season, can reduce the frequency and severity of a viral infection. In fact, if echinacea is taken at the first onset of symptoms, the cold may never develop at all. Once a cold has set in, however, the other remedies in the section may be more beneficial.

Elder Flowers

Elderberry comprises about thirteen species of deciduous shrubs native to North America and Europe. European settlers brought elderberry plants with them to the American colonies. The North American species of elderberry have been used to treat colds, flu, and fevers.

A tea made of elderberry flowers is approved by the German government as a medicine for colds, especially if a cough is present. The flower tea is also used to treat colds and flu in the natural medicine of contemporary Indiana.

Directions: Constituents in the plant's flowers and berries seem to have immunosuppressant properties that help inactivate the influenza virus, halting its spread. Elderberry has been shown to be effective against eight different strains of the flu virus. Drinking too much elderberry tea, however, can leave you feeling nauseous. And, because of a documented diuretic effect, prolonged use may result in hypokalemia, or potassium loss. Avoid the use of elder during pregnancy and lactation.

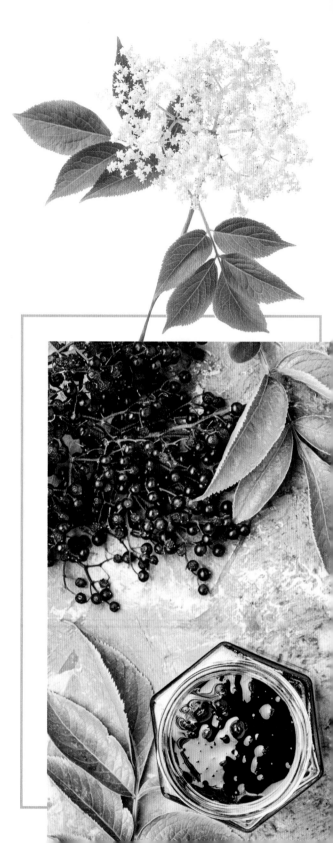

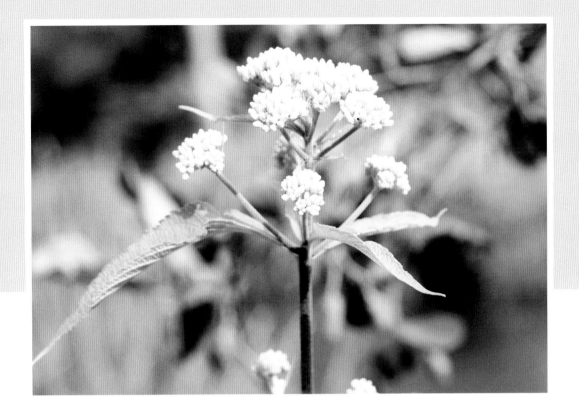

Boneset

The herb boneset (*Eupatorium perfoliatum*) got its name during an influenza epidemic in Pennsylvania in the 1700s. The flu was called "breakbone fever"; the word breakbone referred to the muscle aches and pains that accompanied the virus. Taking the herb, however, proved to "set the bones" and relieve the aches.

The use of boneset for treating colds and flu spread to Europe. Today, some German medical schools continue to study its use. Boneset is frequently prescribed in Germany for treating acute viral infections, for which antibiotic drugs are not effective.

Directions: Constituents have been identified in boneset that are both immune-stimulating and anti-inflammatory. Do not overdo it with boneset, however, because it can induce vomiting if taken in large quantities. It was actually used for that purpose in the 18th and 19th centuries. Boneset is also known to have constituents that are allergenic. Boneset should be avoided during pregnancy and lactation.

Ginger

Ginger tea is a cold remedy that induces sweating, which helps to cool the body during fever.

Directions: *Ginger contains twelve different aromatic anti-inflammatory compounds, including some with aspirin-like effects. Its other proven actions result from its antinauseant and antivertigo properties. Ginger also has carminative (gas relieving), diaphoretic (sweat inducing), and antispasmodic activities.*

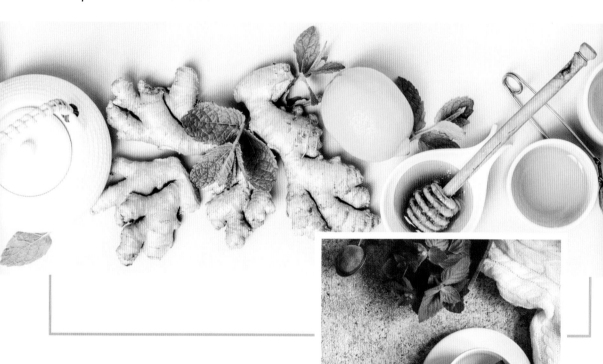

Peppermint

Peppermint *(Mentha piperita)* is a natural remedy used to treat colds. Cornmint *(Mentha arvensis)* is a close relative of the plant and is used for the same purpose.

Directions: *Both plants, when taken as a hot tea, induce sweating and help to cool a fever. Also, the essential oils in the plants, including menthol, act as decongestants when drunk as a tea or inhaled. Peppermint also has antispasmodic and carminative properties.*

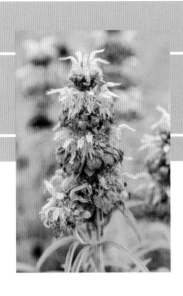

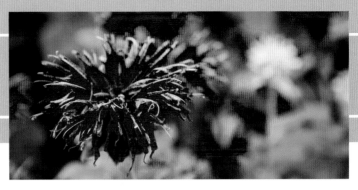

Horsemint-Beebalm Tea

Two closely related species, horsemint (*Monarda punctata*) and beebalm (*Monarda menthaefolia, M. didyma*), are used in natural medicine similarly to the way thyme is used. (Horsemint is native to the eastern United States; beebalm to the Rocky Mountains.)

Directions: Both plants, like thyme, contain high amounts of the constituent thymol, which acts as an expectorant and antiseptic. Both plants also induce sweating and can help cool a fever.

Thyme

Thyme tea (*Thymus vulgaris*) is recommended as a treatment for cold or flu.

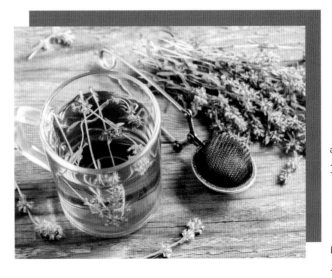

Directions: Thyme taken in the form of a hot tea also induces sweating and helps to cool a fever. Its constituent oil, thymol, is a powerful expectorant and antiseptic. The constituent readily disperses in the steam of a hot tea. Inhaling the steam may effectively spread the thymol throughout the mucous membranes of the upper respiratory tract and bronchial tree. Thus, thymol may help inhibit bacteria, viruses, or fungi from infecting the membranes. Thyme also has mild analgesic and antipyretic (fever reducing) properties.

Fighting Colds, Fevers, and Influenza

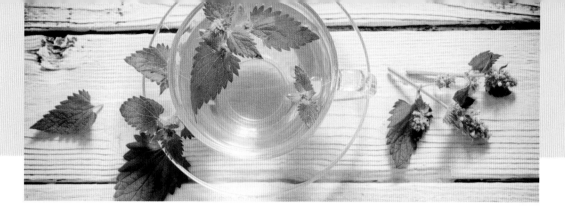

Lemon Balm

Natural remedies enthusiasts have long recommended lemon balm (*Melissa officinalis*) tea for cold and flu. The plant, which is native to southern Europe and northern Africa, now grows throughout North America. Lemon balm has been used as a sweat-inducing herb.

Directions: Lemon balm is approved today by the German government as a medicine for digestive complaints and sleeping disorders, though it is not recommended specifically for colds or flu. Its aromatic oils contain antiviral compounds that may help disinfect the mucous membranes, however. Lemon balm is also a mild sedative and can help relax a restless patient suffering from cold or flu.

Garlic

The recommendation to take garlic for colds comes from New England, the American Southwest, and all the way from China. Garlic has been used for colds, bronchial problems, and fevers in cultures throughout the world since the dawn of written medical history.

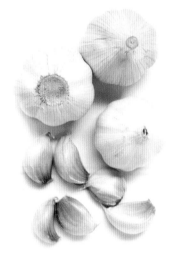

Garlic's constituents are antibacterial, antiviral, and antifungal. Garlic also stimulates the immune system, increasing the body's resistance to invaders. In addition, garlic is an expectorant and induces sweating, helping to reduce fever.

Directions: Garlic has been approved as a medicine for colds and coughs and a variety of other illnesses by the pharmaceutical regulatory commission of the European Union. Garlic can also lower cholesterol and thin the blood. Note that garlic taken in high doses can irritate the stomach.

Onions

Onions are used to treat colds in virtually every folk tradition in North America—whether eaten raw, roasted, or boiled; taken in the form of teas, milk, or wine; worn in a sock or in a bag around the neck; or applied to the chest as a poultice. Wild onions have been used for the same purpose.

Directions: The constituents in onions—the same that cause onion's volatile vapors to burn the eyes—are antimicrobial. Onions also have expectorant qualities, which induce the flow of healthy cleansing mucus. Onions induce sweating as well, helping to cool a fever.

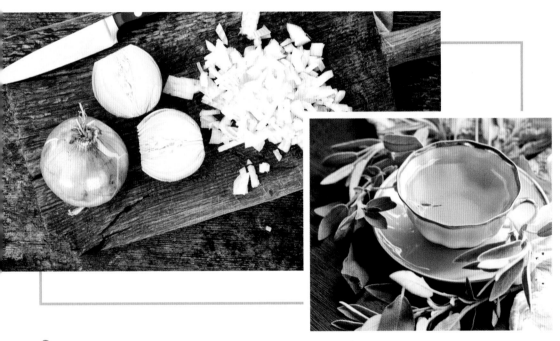

Sage

Sage (*Salvia officinalis*) contains volatile oils, which have been shown to kill viruses in laboratory studies. It specifically kills the rhinovirus, the virus most often responsible for causing colds. Also, because of sage's astringent qualities, it traditionally was used to treat sore throats.

Directions: If you are suffering a sore throat with your cold, hot sage tea may be just the remedy for you. Other documented properties of sage include mild hypotensive effects, anti-inflammatory properties, and analgesic and anticonvulsant effects.

Lemon

The contemporary natural remedies call for drinking "hot lemonade" during a cold or flu. The practice is at least as old as the ancient Romans.

Directions: Lemon juice, like vinegar, is acidic. Drinking it helps to acidify the mucous membranes, making the membranes inhospitable to bacteria or viruses. Lemon oil, which gives the juice its fragrance, is like a pharmacy in itself—it contains antibacterial, antiviral, antifungal, and anti-inflammatory constituents. Five of the constituents are specifically active against the influenza virus. Lemon oil is also an expectorant, increasing the flow of healthy mucous. And lemon is very tasty—its flavor is used to promote compliance in taking cold and flu products.

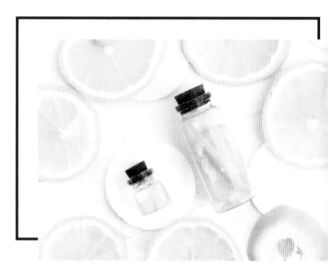

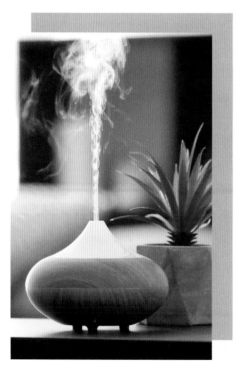

Vaporize It

The contemporary Amish suggest using a vaporizer and adding essential oils to the water, such as pine, cedar, or mint. Many of the aromatic constituents of these plants have antimicrobial properties.

Directions: If you can smell the aroma, then at least a small amount of the constituent has reached your mucous membranes and may assist in killing viruses there. Peppermint oil also contains menthol, which acts as a decongestant. Excessive inhalation can be hazardous to sensitive or allergic young children, however.

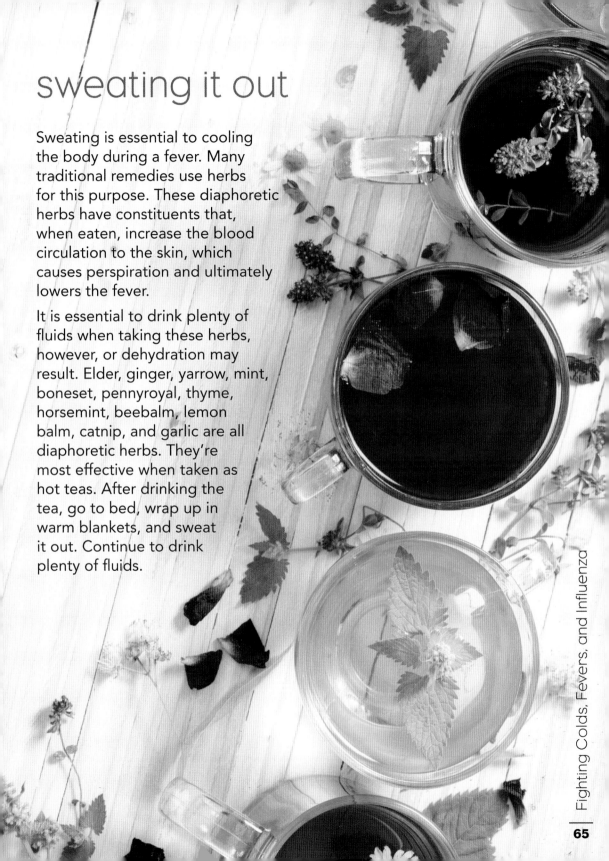

sweating it out

Sweating is essential to cooling the body during a fever. Many traditional remedies use herbs for this purpose. These diaphoretic herbs have constituents that, when eaten, increase the blood circulation to the skin, which causes perspiration and ultimately lowers the fever.

It is essential to drink plenty of fluids when taking these herbs, however, or dehydration may result. Elder, ginger, yarrow, mint, boneset, pennyroyal, thyme, horsemint, beebalm, lemon balm, catnip, and garlic are all diaphoretic herbs. They're most effective when taken as hot teas. After drinking the tea, go to bed, wrap up in warm blankets, and sweat it out. Continue to drink plenty of fluids.

Fighting Colds, Fevers, and Influenza

Chapter 4

BOTANICAL SECRETS FOR CHRONIC CONDITIONS

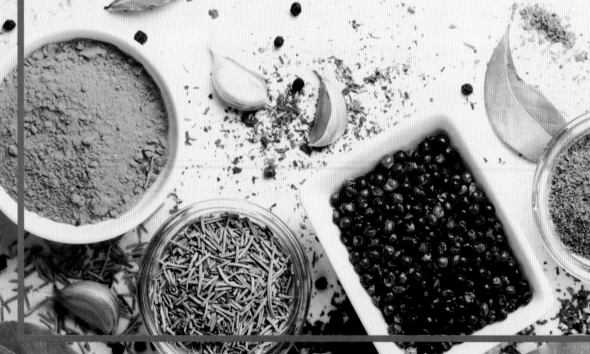

Millions of people suffer from chronic illnesses. Many of these maladies are minor, but others are often debilitating.

But fear not. Some of these conditions—fatigue, allergies, anxiety, arthritis, asthma, headaches, and insomnia—can be managed with a host of natural remedies.

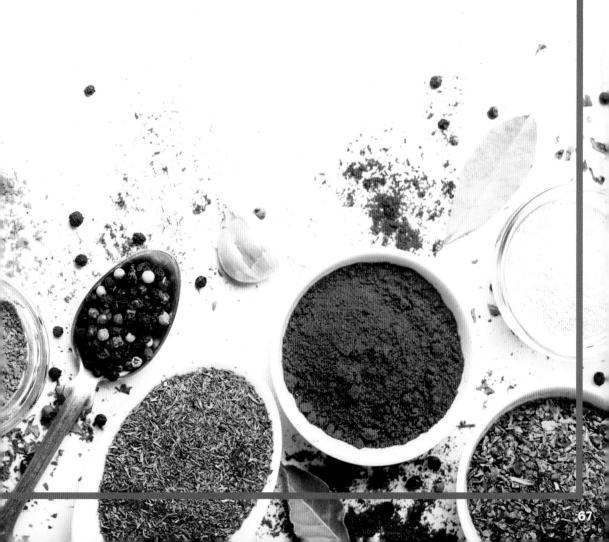

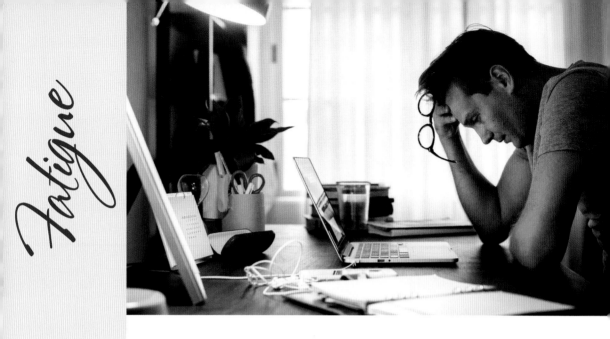

Fatigue

Fatigue may be physical or mental exhaustion, an overwhelming feeling of weariness, or a lack of energy and enthusiasm for even pleasant activities.

Fatigue is a symptom of a vast number of diseases and disorders. More than 10 million people visit their doctors each year complaining of fatigue, making fatigue one of the most common reasons we make a doctor's appointment for a medical checkup. Between one-fourth and one-fifth of all Americans will seek medical advice for severe or chronic fatigue at some point in their professional lives.

Fatigue and tiring rapidly with minimal activity are often among the early signs of an approaching illness. Fatigue is a warning sign of a variety of diseases and disorders, including the common cold, influenza, hepatitis, infectious mononucleosis, and other infectious diseases; heart disease; lung disorders, such as emphysema; some glandular diseases, such as diabetes; and anemia and nutritional deficiencies. Decencies of the minerals magnesium and zinc, the most common mineral deficiencies in the American population affecting more than half of us, may cause fatigue in some people as well.

Deficiencies of chromium, copper, folic acid, manganese, niacin, pantothenic acid, pyridoxine, thiamine, vitamin A, vitamin B12, vitamin C, iron, and potassium may also be responsible. Overwork, either mental or physical, may also cause fatigue, as can psychological disorders or emotional stress. Sugar and caffeine consumption can also result in severe or chronic fatigue in some individuals.

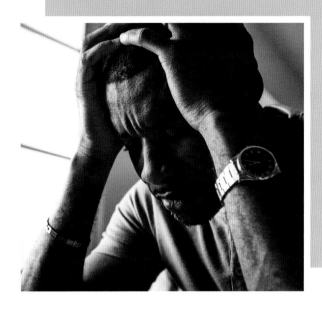

Fatigue is best remedied by treating the physical disorder or psychological problem that is causing it. Some types of fatigue, particularly those due to physical overexertion, can probably be prevented by getting adequate exercise and rest. The average hours of sleep an American gets each night have been on the decline for the last twenty-five years. We now sleep an average of seven hours a night. That's about an hour less than the average optimal amount

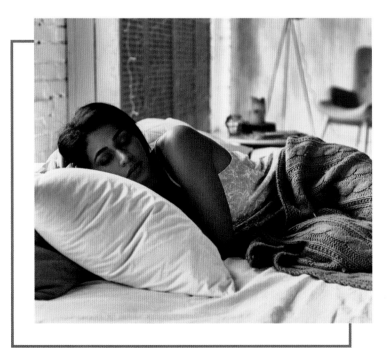

of sleep. A third of Americans sleep less than six hours a night; many of them try to catch up by sleeping more on the weekends. A good alternative to sleeping more at night is to squeeze in naps during the day. Several traditions advocate napping on a regular basis to prevent or treat fatigue.

remedies for fatigue

Betony

A folk source from 1824, listed in Clarence Meyer's *American Folk Medicine*, states that betony *(Stachys officinalis, Betonica officinalis)* is a good remedy for general debility that arises from disturbed digestion. The original source of this remedy was probably an immigrant from Europe, where betony had been used as a tonic since at least the time of the ancient Romans. In fact, the physician to the Emperor Augustus, who lived at the time of Jesus Christ's birth, listed forty-seven different diseases he thought betony would cure. The herb has remained so valued in Italy that a popular expression there advises you to "Sell your coat and buy betony."

Although betony is widely used in natural medicine in Europe even today, it has never been used to any extent by North American schools of medicine or by professional herbalists in North America. Betony is also reputed to be a sedative, and its most common use in European herbalism today is for treating nervous tension, nervous headache, and accompanying exhaustion. Don't confuse this plant with North American betony *(Pedicularis spp.)*, which grows in the mountainous areas of the West. Pedicularis, like Stachys, is a sedative, but does not have the bitter tonic properties.

Directions: Place one tablespoon of betony leaves in a one-pint jar and fill with boiling water. Cover and let cool until the water reaches room temperature. Drink the pint in three doses during the day, twenty minutes before meals, for seven to ten days.

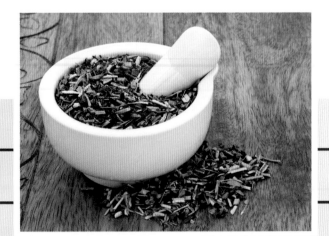

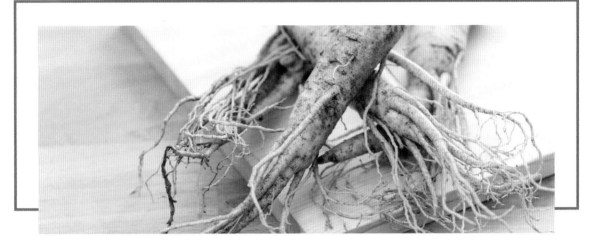

Asian Ginseng

Asian ginseng *(Panax ginseng)* has probably been used in Chinese natural medicine since about 3000 B.C. and remains the most famous and sought-after herbal remedy in Chinese culture. Ginseng is used to restore strength when there is physical weakness or exhaustion resulting from a long-term illness.

Asian ginseng has been used in the natural medicine of Asian communities in North America for at least the last century. In the United States, it entered into mainstream society first through the counterculture movement of the 1960s and 1970s and then through the health food trade and the natural healing movements.

Don't take Asian ginseng unless you are run down, because it can be overstimulating for a person with a normal energy level. Don't take it for chronic fatigue without first getting a thorough medical checkup, because the energy boost from the ginseng may simply temporarily mask the symptoms of a nutritional deficiency or a more serious underlying disease. And don't take ginseng if you also habitually use caffeine. If you begin to experience neck tension, insomnia, increased menstrual flow, or headaches, stop taking ginseng. Prolonged use after experiencing such symptoms can cause high blood pressure.

Directions: Purchase a commercial ginseng product in a reputable herb shop. You'll generally find better quality ginseng there than in a health food store, supermarket, or pharmacy. Don't skimp on price—the more expensive products are usually the better-quality products. Take one to two grams of ginseng powder a day, in two or three doses, for six weeks at a time. Take a two week break every six weeks.

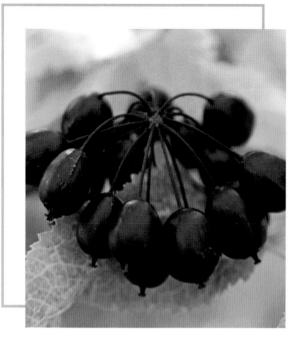

Siberian Ginseng

Siberian ginseng (*Eleutherococcus senticosus, Acanthopanax senticosus*) has been used in Chinese medicine since the birth of Jesus Christ, but its properties as an adaptogen were not clearly identified until after World War II. Russian ginseng researchers investigated the Siberian ginseng plant, looking for a less expensive alternative to Asian ginseng. Both animal and human trials showed that the plant increased response and adaptation to stress. The Siberian ginseng preparation remains a popular medicine in Russia today and is available over-the-counter.

The term Siberian ginseng was invented by marketers trying to sell the product in the United States in the 1970s, hoping to capitalize on the popularity of Asian ginseng. Siberian ginseng thus entered the folklore of North America through health food stores, and is now widely used in every region of the country. It is important to note that the *Eleutherococcus* plant is not actually a "ginseng," however, and it is nowhere near as powerful as Asian ginseng. But it is also less likely to cause overstimulation, insomnia, high blood pressure, or other side effects common to Asian ginseng.

Unfortunately, much of the Siberian ginseng on the market is adulterated. Most American products are also not made according to the specifications of the Russians and are weak by comparison to the Russian products. For the best products, look for a description such as "1:1 extract in 30% alcohol" on the label of the tincture bottle.

Directions: Find a product matching the "1:1" description, and take a dropperful of the tincture three times a day for up to six weeks. Take a two-week break before starting another course of treatment.

An Egg a Day

Folklorist Clarence Meyer's *American Folk Medicine* advises taking an egg a day to restore strength in cases of debility. Deficiencies of several nutrients—including iron, vitamin A, folic acid, riboflavin, and pantothenic acid—may cause fatigue. A single egg contains significant amounts of these nutrients.

Directions: Beat a raw egg, flavor it with a little sugar or honey, and drink it. If the texture is not appetizing, blend the egg in a glass of milk and drink it that way. (Note: A raw egg may be contaminated with salmonella and should be cooked before eating.)

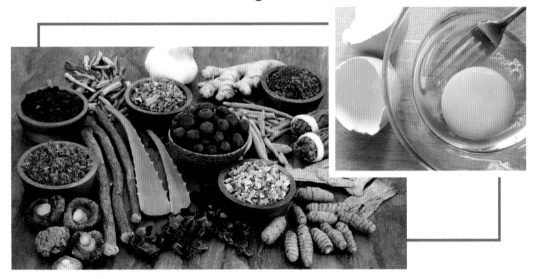

Adaptogens

An entire class of Chinese herbs—ginseng being the most famous of them—are used to restore the weary. These herbs and their beneficial actions were made more accessible to Westerners when Russian researchers investigated them in the decades after World War II. In fact, it was the Russians who coined the term adaptogen. An adaptogen helps you "adapt" to different kinds of stress, whether from cold weather, overwork, or staying up at night with a crying baby. The Russians verified this adaptogen property in Asian ginseng, Siberian ginseng, schizandra berries, and several other herbs. These plants are now popular in various other communities throughout the United States as well. In fact, you can purchase various kinds of ginseng today in most pharmacies and supermarkets.

pick-me-up combo

-8 drops lemon oil
-2 drops eucalyptus oil
-2 drops peppermint oil
-1 drop cinnamon leaf oil
-1 drop cardamom oil (expensive, so optional)
-2 ounces vegetable oil

Directions: Combine the ingredients. Use as a massage oil, add 2 teaspoons to your bath, or add 1 teaspoon to a footbath. Without the vegetable oil, this combination can be used in an aromatherapy diffuser, simmering pan of water, or a potpourri cooker, or it can be added to 2 ounces of water for an air spray. The cardamom oil is optional, but, oh, does it enhance this massage oil! Use it as often as you like.

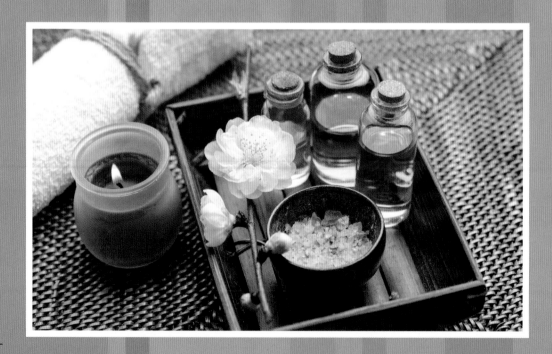

Allergies & Hay Fever

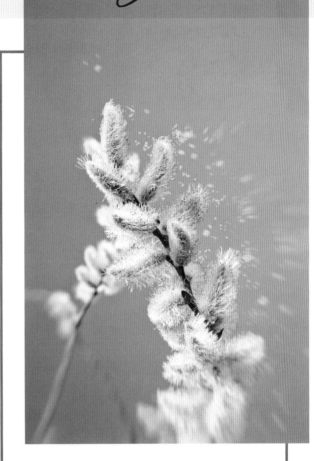

Our bodies are constantly assaulted by substances from the environment, in the form of bacteria, viruses, molds, dust, pollen, and other potential invaders. Our immune system reacts to these substances through chemical and blood responses that attempt to neutralize the invaders or eliminate them from the body. One specialized immune response is the allergic reaction, in which specialized cells stimulated by an invading substance release the chemical histamine into the tissues. The histamine can cause swelling, increased circulation, and sneezing, actions designed to isolate the invader, eliminate it, or render it harmless. An allergic reaction can occur in the respiratory tract, skin, or eyes.

An allergic reaction is a healthy, protective response to an invader, but, in some individuals, the body overreacts, and the uncomfortable reactions are far in excess of what is necessary to neutralize the offending substance. The most noticeable allergic symptoms are sneezing, red swollen eyes, shortness of breath (in asthma), rashes, eczema, or the swelling that accompanies insect bites and stings.

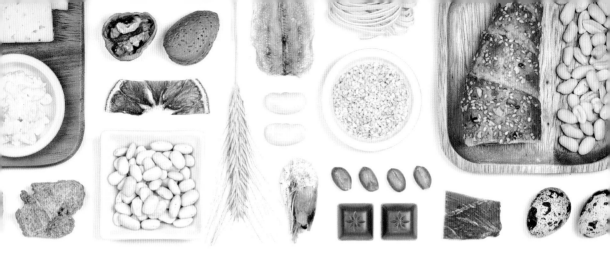

Food allergies can also cause symptoms in the digestive tract, but these are usually less noticeable to the sufferer than the external reactions above. The worst type of allergic reaction—called anaphylaxis—is an overwhelming allergic reaction that can lead to death. Any swelling of the airways or shortness of breath during an allergic reaction is an emergency.

Allergies tend to run in families, so some people may be genetically predisposed to having them. It has also been suggested that nutrient deficiencies common in the modern diet may also contribute to allergies. Dietary deficiencies of calcium and magnesium, which are common deficiencies in Americans, can also increase allergic symptoms. Studies have shown that the body's stores of vitamin C correlate inversely with the release of histamine during an allergy attack, so an abundant dietary intake of vitamin C may reduce allergy symptoms. Omega-3 essential fatty acids, such as those that occur naturally in cold-water fish and wild game, are also natural anti-inflammatory substances that can reduce the intensity of allergies.

Antihistamine drugs and avoidance of allergens are the most common conventional treatments for symptoms of allergy. The drugs work by blocking the effects of histamine in the tissues, but they do not reduce its release. Desensitization involves medical treatments where small amounts of an allergen may also be injected into the body in the form of allergy shots in order to reduce the body's reaction to it. The folk remedies listed here do not address the cause of allergies but may reduce allergy symptoms through their astringent or anti-inflammatory actions.

remedies for allergies & hay fever

Horseradish

Horseradish (*Armoracia rusticana*), popular today as a sushi condiment, was an early American remedy for hay fever. If you've used it as a condiment, you're probably well aware that it causes watery eyes and a burning sensation in the sinus tissues. These effects are due to its constituent allyl isothiocyanate, which is related chemically to the substances in watercress, red radish, and brown and yellow mustard. Scientific studies have shown that allyl isothiocyanate has decongestant and antiasthmatic properties.

Directions: *Purchase grated horseradish as a condiment. Take a dose of ¼ teaspoon during a congestive hay fever attack. You can take horseradish as often as desired—or as much as you can stand!*

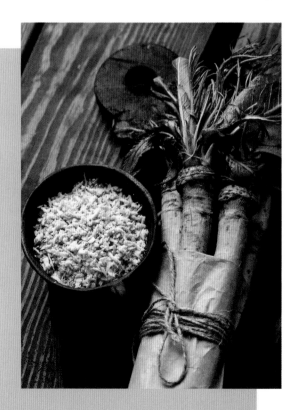

An alternate method, if you have access to fresh horseradish root, comes from an old New England remedy. Take fresh horseradish roots, wash, and blend, skin and all, in your blender. Fill half of a one-quart jar with the ground roots. Add enough vinegar to cover the roots, and close the jar tightly. Store the jar at room temperature. When suffering a hay fever attack, remove the cap, place your nose into the jar, and sniff or inhale. (Do this carefully at first to avoid irritating your nose and eyes.) Quickly replace the cap to keep the remaining aromatic substances from escaping.

Horsemint

In the medicine of southern Appalachia, horsemint (*Monarda punctata*) is a traditional treatment for hay fever. Horsemint may be inhaled, or you can drink it as a simple tea. Horsemint is not readily available in stores today, but its anti-allergic constituent is probably the essential oil thymol. Scientific studies have shown that thymol reduces swelling in the bronchial tract, relaxes the trachea, and acts as an anti-inflammatory and mild antibacterial. The kitchen spice thyme also contains large amounts of this aromatic oil and can be substituted for horsemint.

Directions: *Place ½ ounce of ground thyme in a one-pint jar and cover with boiling water. Close the jar tightly and let the mixture cool for half an hour. Remove the lid and inhale, taking a few deep breaths. Do this as needed throughout the day.*

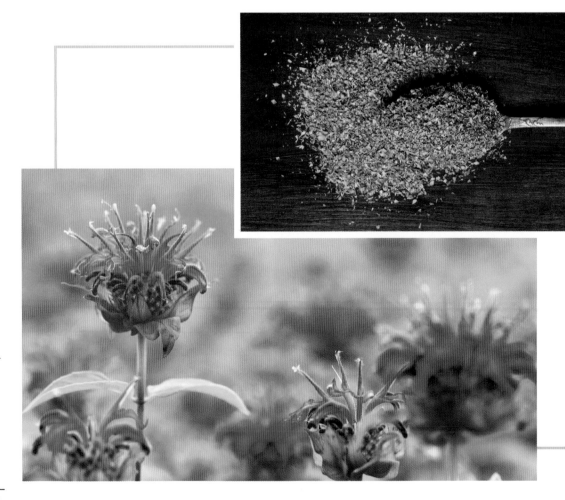

Chamomile & Thyme Oil

German immigrants inhaled the fumes of chamomile tea (*Matricaria recutita*) to treat bouts of hay fever. In contemporary German naturopathic medicine, three to five drops of the essential oil of thyme is added to chamomile tea for the same purpose. Chamomile contains the essential oil azulene and related oils that are anti-inflammatory and anti-allergic, as well as the oil alpha-bisabolol, which is also an anti-inflammatory.

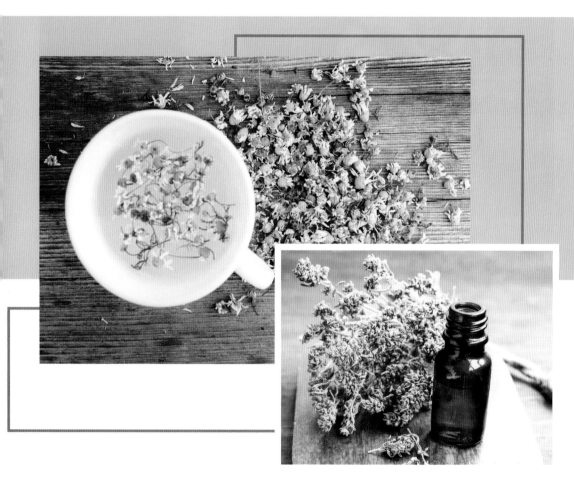

Directions: Place ½ ounce of chamomile flowers in a one-quart jar. Fill two thirds of the jar with boiling water. Add three to five drops of essential oil of thyme. Cover and let cool for half an hour. Open the lid and inhale the fumes, taking a few deep breaths. Repeat as desired throughout the day. (Be careful of inhaling flower dust, because the pollen causes allergies in some people.)

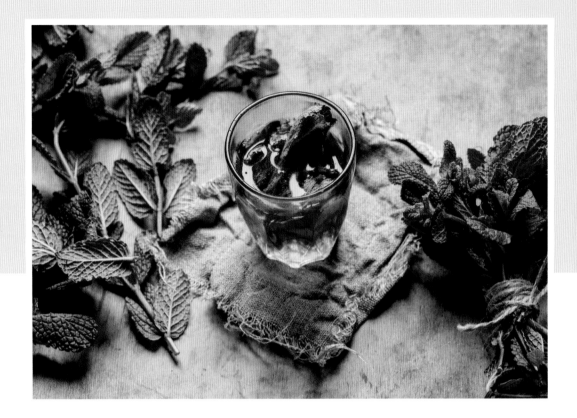

Mint Teas

Inhaling, drinking, or washing affected skin areas with mint teas can be accredited in this country to the natural medicine of the Seneca Indians. The plants used to make the teas are peppermint *(Mentha piperita)* and spearmint *(Mentha spicata)*.

When consumed as a tea or inhaled, the essential oils in the mints act as a decongestant. When applied to the skin, the menthol in peppermint and cornmint produces a cooling sensation and reduces itching. (Spearmint contains little menthol, however, so it does not have this effect on the skin.) All three of the mints contain other anti-inflammatory and mild antibacterial constituents.

Directions: Place ½ ounce of dried mint leaves in a one-quart jar. Fill two thirds of the jar with boiling water and cover the jar tightly. Let cool for half an hour. Strain and drink. The tea's fumes will also help relieve congestion.

Eyebright

The use of eyebright (*Euphrasia officinalis*) to treat allergies in the eastern United States dates back at least 150 years and may have had its roots among German immigrants. At the turn of the century, Eclectic physicians also used eyebright to treat allergy symptoms among their patients. During the same period, the pharmaceutical companies Parke Davis and Eli Lilly sold eyebright allergy preparations to the public. Eyebright is still used today in Appalachia as a natural remedy for allergies.

Eyebright contains the constituents caffeic acid and ferulic acid, both of which have an anti-inflammatory effect. The caffeic acid also has specific antihistamine effects.

Directions: You can purchase eyebright tincture in a health food store or herb shop. Take a dropperful every three to four hours during the height of allergy season.

Another option is to make your own tincture. Place two ounces of dried eyebright leaves in a one-pint jar and fill the jar with grain alcohol or 100 proof gin or vodka. Cover the jar and let it stand in a cool, dark place for three weeks, shaking the jar each day. After three weeks, strain and store the solution in the refrigerator. Take as directed above.

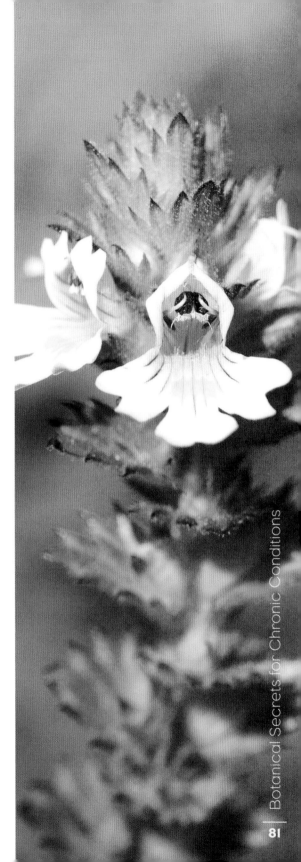

Anxiety

Everyone experiences some anxiety. Anxiety helps us stay alert and adapt to the ever-changing demands of our environment. Anxiety is really the body's "early warning system" against harm. When we feel danger, the alarm goes off to warn us and prevent injury. The body responds immediately to the alarm emotionally, physically, and behaviorally. Emotionally, we may feel fear, doom, or anger. Physically, our hearts race, muscles tense, breathing becomes rapid, and palms and feet start to sweat. We respond behaviorally by getting ready to fight or flee from danger.

The anxiety warning system works fine when there's clear and present danger, but anxiety can become a problem for people when they perceive harmless situations as threatening.

There is no single reason why some people experience episodes of chronic anxiety. Some of these individuals will benefit from visiting a psychotherapist. Any physical change, such as illness, can also cause anxiety. Anemia, diabetes, premenstrual syndrome, menopause, thyroid disorder, hypoglycemia, pulmonary disease, endocrine tumors, and other conditions can cause anxiety symptoms. Other individuals simply need to improve their nutrition and lifestyle—anxiety can be the symptom of several nutrient deficiencies or lifestyle habits that are common in modern society.

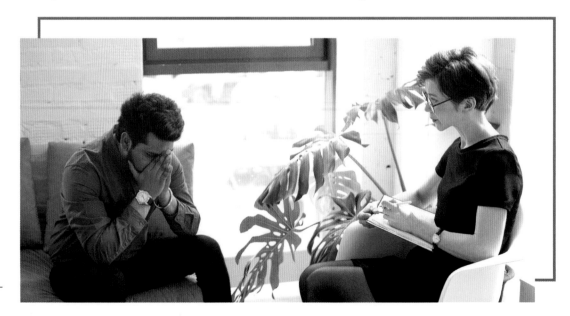

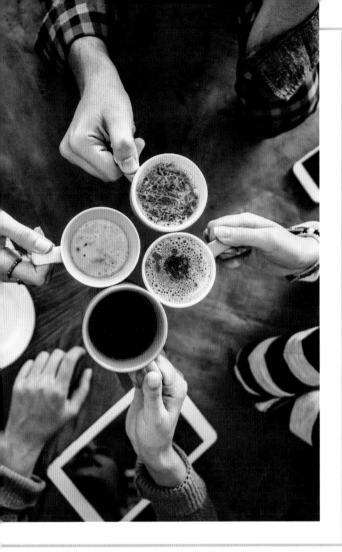

One of the most commonly overlooked causes of anxiety and nervousness in modern life is related to caffeine consumption. Even moderate amounts of caffeine can create nervous symptoms severe enough to earn a diagnosis of chronic anxiety—and a subsequent prescription of sedative drugs or referral to a therapist.

You don't need to take a lot of caffeine in order to experience these symptoms. Some of us can get away with drinking a few cups of coffee every day, but others can develop the symptoms of caffeinism even from a small amount.

One scientific theory suggests that anxiety is closely associated with the balance of the substances lactate and pyruvate in the body. These two substances are associated with energy production within the cells, and high lactate levels may cause anxiety. Alcohol, caffeine, and sugar all increase lactate levels, and the B-vitamins niacin and thiamine and the mineral magnesium all lower it. Deficiencies of the B-vitamins as well as omega-3 fatty acids, such as occur naturally in fish and wild game, may thus contribute to anxiety.

Conventional treatment of anxiety is primarily with drugs of the benzodiazepine class, such as Valium and Xanax. Anxiety patients are often treated by psychotherapists as well. Here are some natural remedies you can try to help ease feelings of stress and anxiety.

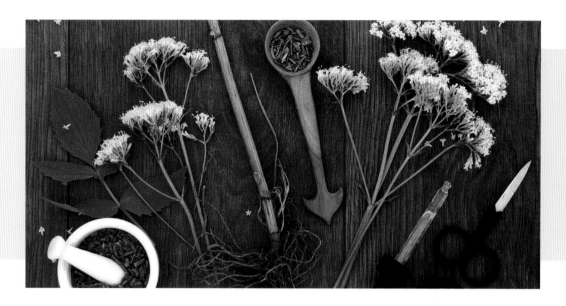

remedies for anxiety

Valerian

In natural medicine traditions, valerian is considered a universal sedative. The Greeks used valerian as a relaxant and antispasmodic. The herb was also used in the medicine of India and Japan. Today, naturalists use varieties of the plant native to their regions.

Valeriana of cinalis, the European variety of the plant, was brought to the eastern colonies by immigrants for cultivation. It has subsequently become native in the eastern United States. Valerian is recognized today as an official medicine for nervousness and anxiety by the German government. Valerian has proven to be as effective as the sedative Valium in some clinical trials, although it has no relationship chemically to that drug. Valerian can cause stimulation rather than sedation in some individuals, however, especially those with "hot" constitutions, as might be indicated by feelings of warmth, by red flushed cheeks, and by desire for cool drinks.

Directions: Place two to three teaspoons of dried chopped valerian root in a cup and cover with boiling water. Cover the cup and let stand for fifteen minutes. Drink two to three cups a day for up to three weeks. Individuals who use valerian for longer than three weeks, or who use valerian to help them get to sleep, can ultimately develop lethargy or hangover effects.

Valerian-Hop Tea

German immigrants of the late 18th century treated nervousness with a mixture of equal portions of valerian (*Valeriana officinalis*) and hop (*Humulus lupulus*). Commercial combinations of these two herbs are still popular in Germany today.

Directions: Mix equal amounts by volume of dried and chopped valerian root and hop in a bowl. Place one tablespoon of the mixture in a cup and fill the cup with boiling water. Cover the cup and let stand for twenty minutes. Strain and drink three cups a day. Take nightly for up to three weeks.

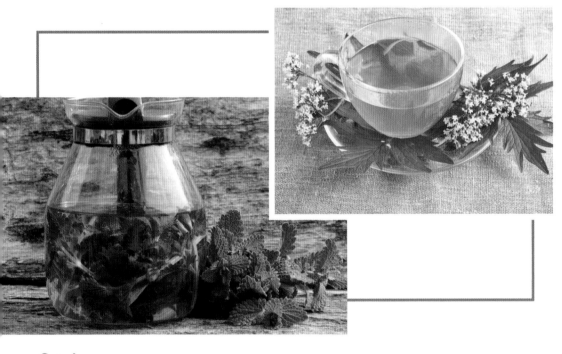

Catnip

Catnip tea has been used as a popular sleep aid in America since the arrival of European immigrants in New England. The Onondaga and Cayuga tribes used it to calm restless children, and European New Englanders gave it to adults for nervous disorders, including nervous breakdown.

Directions: Place one to three teaspoons of the dried herb in a cup and cover with boiling water. Cover the cup and let stand for ten minutes. Strain and drink three cups a day. Use as needed.

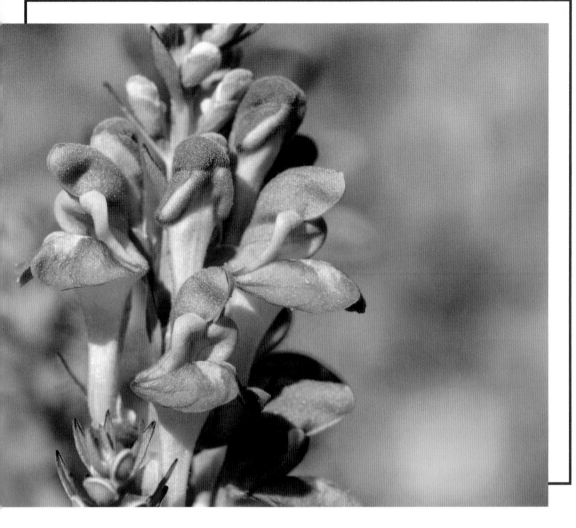

Skullcap

More than a hundred species of skullcap (*Scutellaria* spp.) grow throughout the world. North American varieties of the herb were used by Native American tribes such as the Penobscot, Iroquois, and Cherokee to treat diarrhea and heart disease and to promote menstruation and eliminate afterbirth. Skullcap received its common name, mad dog weed, in the 18th century, when the herb was widely prescribed as a cure for rabies. It is still used today in Appalachian folk medicine as a sedative. The suspected medicinal constituents are flavonoids and an essential oil.

Directions: Put two teaspoonfuls of dried skullcap leaves in a cup and fill with boiling water. Cover and steep for fifteen minutes. Strain and drink three to four cups a day as needed.

Rosemary

European and Spanish immigrants brought the herb rosemary *(Rosmarinus officinalis)* with them to cultivate in the New World. Rosemary was later used by early Californians to rid the body of "evil spirits" or to treat epilepsy, which in ancient times was considered to be a form of possession.

Rosemary has long been used in European and Chinese medicine to calm the nerves. Medical experts in the United States continue to recommend rosemary to treat nervous conditions. Rosemary's analgesic and antispasmodic properties are also recognized by the German government; the herb is used there as an official medical treatment for spastic conditions, including epilepsy.

Directions: Add one or two teaspoons of the dried herb to a cup and fill the cup with boiling water. Cover the cup and let it stand ten minutes. Strain and drink two to three cups a day as needed.

Vervain

Vervain *(Verbena spp.)* has long been used as a sedative among residents of the Southwest and Appalachia. It has been used in European medicine since antiquity for the same purposes. Its constituent verbenalin promotes relaxation. Vervain is claimed to be especially useful for recovery from the exhaustion of long-term stress.

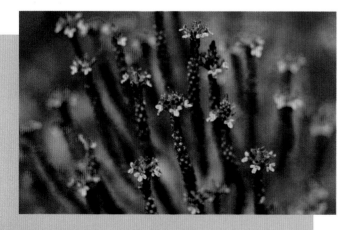

Directions: Add one or two teaspoons of the dried herb to a cup and fill with boiling water. Cover the cup and let it stand ten minutes. Strain and drink two to three cups a day as needed.

Passion Flower

Of nineteen passion flower species worldwide, eight have been used as sedatives by various cultures. Passion flower *(Passiflora incarnata)* is native from Florida to Texas and may also be found as far north as Missouri. The herb is abundant in South America; it's long-time use as a sedative there is recorded in Brazilian medicine.

The passion flower species *P. incarnata* was introduced into American professional medicine in 1840 after medical doctors in Mississippi experimented with it and demonstrated its sedative effects. Thereafter the herb was mainly used by doctors of the Eclectic school. Passion flower is still popularly used as a sedative among residents of southern Appalachia and among the Amish. The herb is also widely cultivated in Europe for medicinal purposes; it is approved by the German government as a sedative medicine. Passion flower is a gentle sedative and is often combined with other plants. Most likely, its active constituent is an alkaloid, called passiflorine (or harmane).

Directions: Place one heaping teaspoon of dried passion flower in a cup, fill the cup with boiling water, cover, and steep for ten minutes. Strain and drink as needed.

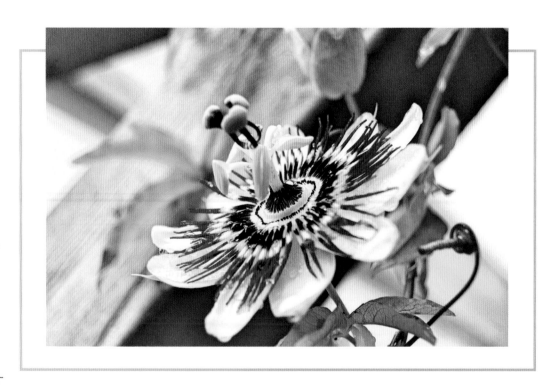

Asafoetida

Asafoetida *(Ferula assafoetida)*, a relative of garlic and onions, is a traditional medicine from Asia. Its usage as a calming agent probably arrived in North America by way of immigrating European physicians. The Eclectic physicians of the 1920s used asafoetida as a sedative. The herb is still used today in Appalachian herbalism to treat nervousness and mental stress.

Asafoetida has at least two sedative constituents, including ferulic acid, which is analgesic, antispasmodic, and acts as a muscle relaxant, and valeric acid, which induces sleep, relaxes muscle, and acts as a sedative.

Directions: Stir ¼ teaspoon of asafoetida powder into a little warm water and drink. Do this two or three times a day. If asafoetida begins to cause heartburn, reduce the dose or try another sedative. Asafoetida has a strong, disagreeable garlic-like odor.

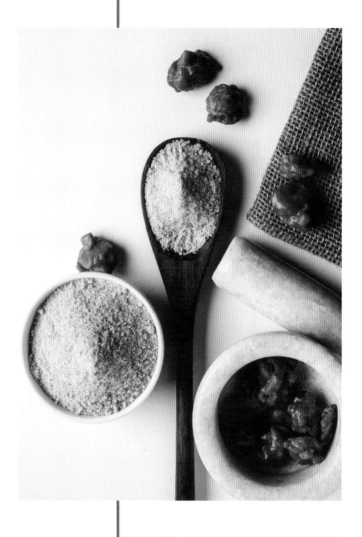

Motherwort

Motherwort is a mild relaxing agent often recommended by herbalists to reduce anxiety and depression and treat nervousness, insomnia, heart palpitations, and rapid heart rate. Motherwort (*Leonurus cardiaca*) has been used in Europe since antiquity as a sedative and to treat menstrual irregularities. It probably came to North America with physicians among the British colonists. American Indian tribes later adopted the herb's medicinal uses.

Today, in Germany, motherwort is an approved medicine for treating anxiety. It is also used in contemporary Chinese medicine for the same purpose. The herb contains a chemical called leonurine, which may encourage uterine contractions, however. Thus, you will want to avoid motherwort if you are pregnant or trying to conceive a child.

Directions: *Place one to two teaspoons of motherwort herb in a cup and fill the cup with boiling water. Cover the cup and let stand for ten to fifteen minutes. Strain and drink. The tea's taste is bitter. Don't drink more than two to three cups a day.*

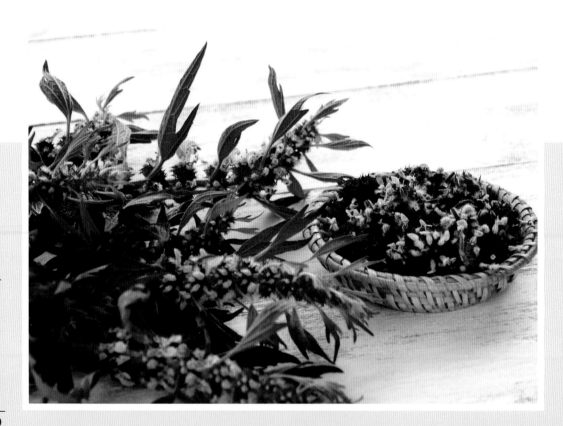

Arthritis

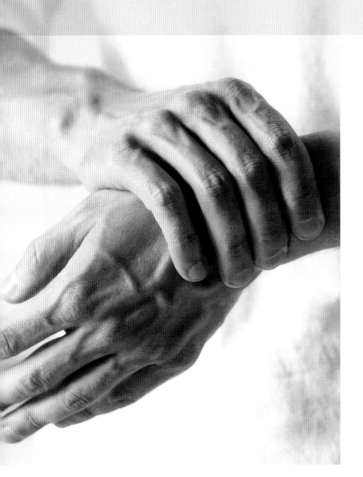

In a nutshell, arthritis means "inflammation of the joints." Rheumatism is an old medical term that was used to describe inflammation of either joints or muscles. Rheum was thought to be a watery mucus-like secretion, sometimes brought on by cold weather. Joint or muscle pain was thought to be caused by such secretions trapped in the tissues. Although the concept is not far from the truth—inflammation is usually accompanied by swelling and a build-up of fluid—the modern explanation of arthritis is much more precise.

Today's medical experts suggest there are at least twenty-three varieties of arthritis, including rheumatoid arthritis and osteoarthritis, the two most common types. With osteoarthritis—sometimes called degenerative joint disease, or DJD—there is a gradual wearing away of cartilage in the joints. Healthy cartilage is the elastic tissue that lines and cushions the joints and allows bones to move smoothly against one another. When this cartilage deteriorates, the bones rub together, causing pain and swelling. Permanent damage and stiffness of the joints is possible.

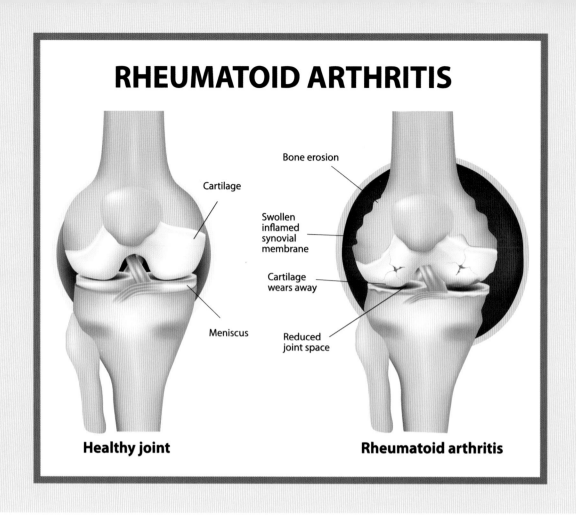

RHEUMATOID ARTHRITIS

Cartilage

Meniscus

Healthy joint

Bone erosion

Swollen inflamed synovial membrane

Cartilage wears away

Reduced joint space

Rheumatoid arthritis

Rheumatoid arthritis can attack at any age. This form of arthritis affects all the connective tissues, as well as other organs. The precise cause of rheumatoid arthritis is unknown. Some researchers believe that a virus triggers the disease, causing an autoimmune response whereby the body attacks its own tissues. However, evidence for this theory is inconclusive. What is confirmed is the progression of the condition. First, the synovium (the thin membrane that lines and lubricates the joint) becomes inflamed. The inflammation eventually destroys the cartilage. As scar tissue gradually replaces the damaged cartilage, the joint becomes misshapen and rigid. Rheumatoid arthritis may damage the heart, lungs, nerves, eyes, and joints.

A medical examination and diagnosis are required to identify the cause and nature of any chronic joint or muscular pain. Other "rheumatic" diseases include arthralgia (pain in a joint), fibrositis ("muscular rheumatism"), and synovitis (inflammation of the joint membrane). There is no simple cure for arthritis. Conventional treatment for chronic joint pain is to use drugs to suppress the inflammation in order to reduce pain and also prevent tissue destruction. Usually, simple aspirin-related pain medications, called nonsteroidal anti-inflammatory drugs (NSAIDs), are first prescribed. Corticosteroids may be prescribed for more serious illness, especially when tissue destruction is evident. In about fifteen percent of rheumatoid arthritis cases, these measures are ineffective, and stronger substances are used. Oral or injectable gold may prove helpful in treating rheumatoid arthritis. Some drugs usually used for cancer treatment may also be helpful.

Alternative physicians usually treat arthritis by recommending short fasts, screening for food allergies, recommending avoidance of processed foods, introducing fish and fish oils to the diet as well as anti-inflammatory herbal and nutritional supplements, and using natural methods to improve digestion. Alternative physicians may also recommend the substance glucosamine sulfate, which provides natural building blocks for cartilage, as a dietary supplement for those suffering from osteoarthritis. Scientific studies have suggested that supplementation with B vitamins, vitamin E, and some minerals (including the trace elements copper and selenium) may also improve the disease. On the other hand, studies have shown that nightshade vegetables—potatoes, tomatoes, bell peppers, and chili peppers—may provoke joint pain.

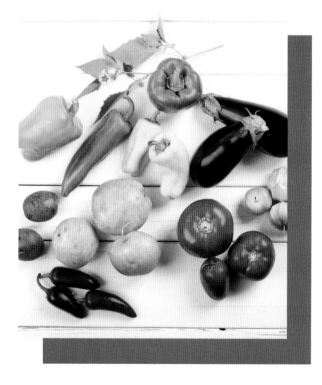

Very few of the herbs or foods recommended as a natural remedy for treating arthritis have been tested clinically for anti-inflammatory effects. Many of these herbs and foods contain plant constituents for which such effects are known, however.

remedies for arthritis

Celery

The remedy of eating raw or cooked celery seeds (*Apium graveolens*) or large amounts of the celery plant to treat rheumatism arrived in North America with the British and German immigrants. Using celery to treat rheumatism persists today in North American professional herbalism. Various parts of the celery plant contain more than twenty-five different anti-inflammatory compounds.

Directions: Place one teaspoon of celery seeds in a cup. Fill the cup with boiling water. Cover and let stand for fifteen minutes. Strain and drink three cups a day during an acute attack.

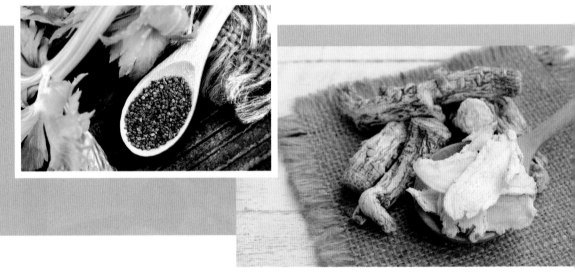

Angelica

Angelica (*Angelica archangelica*), an herb that has been used in European folk medicine since antiquity, can be used to treat arthritis. The Western variety of angelica has twelve anti-inflammatory constituents, ten antispasmodic (muscle relaxant) constituents, and five anodyne (pain-relieving) ones. The Chinese sometimes use their native variety of the plant (*Angelica sinensis*) for the same purpose.

Directions: Place one tablespoon of the cut roots of either species of angelica in one pint of water and bring to a boil. Cover and boil for two minutes. Remove from heat and let stand, covered, until the water cools to room temperature. Strain and drink the tea in three doses during the day for two to three weeks at a time. Then, take a break for seven to ten days and start the treatment again if desired.

Rosemary

Clarence Meyer suggests drinking rosemary tea to treat arthritis. The same remedy is used in the contemporary natural medicine of the Coahuila tribe in Mexico. Rosemary has been used to relieve pain and spasms. The plant's leaves contain four anti-inflammatory substances—carnosol, oleanolic acid, rosmarinic acid, and ursolic acid. Carnosol acts on the same anti-inflammatory pathways as both steroids and aspirin, oleanolic acid has been marketed as an antioxidant in China, rosmarinic acid acts as an anti-inflammatory, and ursolic acid, which makes up about four percent of the plant by weight, has been shown to have antiarthritic effects in animal trials.

Directions: *Put ½ ounce of rosemary leaves in a one-quart canning jar and fill the jar with boiling water. Cover tightly and let stand for thirty minutes. Drink a cup of the hot tea before going to bed and have another cupful in the morning before breakfast. Do this for two to three weeks, and then take a break for seven to ten days before starting the treatment again.*

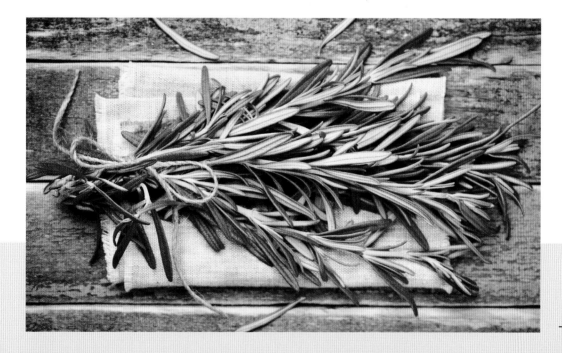

Wintergreen

Wintergreen (*Gaulteria procumbens*) was used to treat arthritis by the Delaware, Menominee, Ojibwa, Potawatomi, and Iroquois tribes. The plant was accepted in the United States as an official medicine for arthritis in 1820; it is still included—in the form of wintergreen oil— in the *United States Pharmacopoeia* today. The chief active pain-relieving constituent in wintergreen is methyl salicylate. This compound can be toxic when consumed in concentrated wintergreen oil, even when applied to the skin, so, if you want to use this plant, stick with using the dried herb. (Aspirin was developed as a safer alternative to methyl salicylate.)

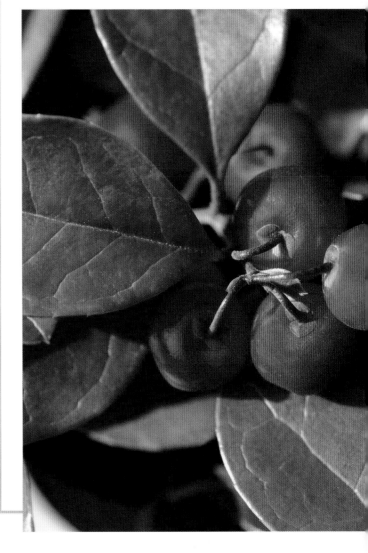

Directions: Place one or two teaspoons of dried wintergreen leaves in a cup and cover with boiling water. Cover and let steep for fifteen minutes. Strain and drink three cups a day. Do this for two to three weeks, and then take a break for seven to ten days before starting again.

Black Cohosh

An American Indian treatment for arthritis, in both the Seneca and Cherokee tribes, involved using the root of black cohosh (*Cimicifuga racemosa*). White settlers in the eastern states eventually adopted the plant's use, as did the Eclectic physicians of the last century. There are five species in the Cimicifuga genus worldwide that have been used to treat rheumatism. Black cohosh contains aspirin-like substances as well as other anti-inflammatory and antispasmodic constituents.

Directions: Simmer one teaspoon of black cohosh root in one cup of boiling water for twenty minutes. Strain and drink the tea in two divided doses during the day. Do this for two to three weeks. Take a break for seven to ten days before starting the treatment again.

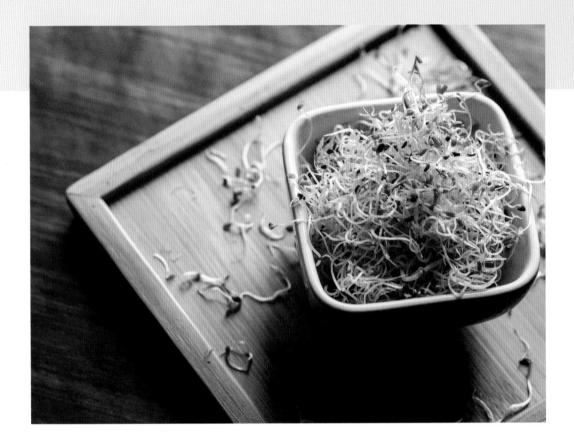

Alfalfa

Alfalfa *(Medicago sativa)* is often promoted in health food stores as an arthritis remedy—in the form of capsulated alfalfa powder. Alfalfa contains L-canavanine, however, an amino acid that can cause symptoms that are similar to those of systemic lupus, an autoimmune disease that can also cause joint pain. Some scientific studies show that these symptoms can occur in both animals and humans as a result of eating alfalfa. Thus, the remedy below is best taken in the form of a tea rather than powder; the amino acid is not present to any significant amount in alfalfa tea. Alfalfa tea is rich with nutritive minerals. It is a recommended natural remedy for arthritis in southern Appalachia.

Directions: Place one ounce of alfalfa tea in a pot. Cover with one quart of water and boil for thirty minutes. Strain and drink the quart throughout the day. Do this for two to three weeks, and then take a break for seven to ten days before starting again.

Sesame Seeds

A remedy for arthritis from Chinese medicine is to eat sesame seeds. A half ounce of the seeds contains about 4 grams of essential fatty acids, 175 milligrams of calcium, 64 milligrams of magnesium, and, notably, .73 milligrams of copper. Increased copper intake may be important during arthritis attacks because the body's requirements go up during inflammation.

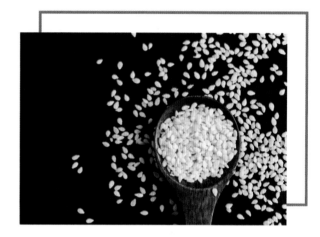

Directions: Grind up ½ ounce of sesame seeds in a coffee grinder and sprinkle on your food at mealtime. You can use this treatment for as long as you like.

Mustard Plaster

Perhaps the most famous of the counterirritant treatments for arthritis in the mustard plaster. This treatment is used throughout Europe and also in Appalachia and China. The irritating substance in mustard is allyl-isothiocyanate, which is related to the acrid substances in garlic and onions. This constituent is not activated, however, until the seeds are crushed and mixed with some liquid. Only then does the mustard produce the irritation necessary for the counterirritant effect.

Directions: Crush the seeds of white or brown mustard (Brassica alba, Brassica juncea) or grind them in a seed grinder. Moisten the mixture with

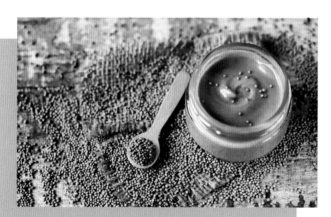

vinegar, then sprinkle with flour. Spread the mixture on a cloth. Place the cloth, poultice side down, on the skin. Leave on for no more than twenty minutes. Remove if the poultice becomes uncomfortable. After removing the poultice, wash the affected area.

Hot Peppers

Cayenne pepper (*Capsicum* spp.) appears in counterirritant potions in China, the American Southwest, and throughout Ohio, Indiana, and Illinois. External and internal use of cayenne pepper was a key element of Thomsonian herbalism, which was popular throughout rural New England and the Midwest in the early 1800s. Cayenne works by reducing substance P, a chemical that carries pain messages from the skin's nerve endings, so it reduces pain when applied topically. Try this simple cayenne liniment.

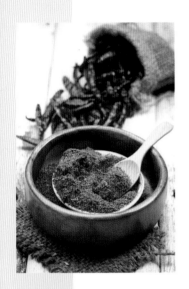

Directions: Place one ounce of cayenne pepper in one quart of rubbing alcohol (a poison not for internal use). Let stand for three weeks, shaking the bottle each day. Then, using a cloth, apply to the affected area during acute attacks of pain. Leave the solution in place for ten to twenty minutes, then wipe clean.

Ginseng Liquor

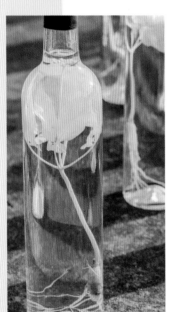

The Iroquois tribe used American ginseng (*Panax quinquefolius*) as a treatment for rheumatism. Today, the Chinese use the herb for the same purpose. Be sure to use American ginseng, however, not Asian ginseng (*Panax ginseng*); Asian ginseng can actually aggravate the pain of arthritis. Ginseng contains constituents called ginsenosides, which have a variety of pharmacological actions. Both the American and Asian varieties of the plant are classified as adaptogens, meaning that they increase the body's ability to handle a wide variety of stresses. The Iroquois Indians made a tea of the plant's roots and added whiskey.

Directions: Chop three and a half ounces of ginseng and place in one quart of liquor like vodka. Let the mixture stand for five to six weeks in a cool dark place, turning the container frequently. Strain and take one ounce of the liquid after dinner or before bedtime every night for up to three months. Then, take a break for two weeks before starting the treatment again.

Hop Tea

Hop is native to Europe and can be found in vacant fields and along rivers there. The Pilgrims brought hop (*Humulus lupulus*) to Massachusetts, and it quickly spread south to Virginia. The hop plant contains at least twenty-two constituents that have anti-inflammatory activities, including several that act through the same cellular mechanisms as steroid drugs. Four constituents have antispasmodic properties, and ten may act as sedatives. Today, a popular remedy for rheumatism in Mexico and the American Southwest is hop tea.

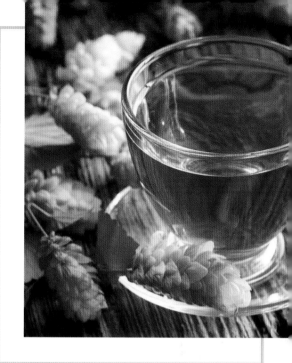

Directions: Place two or three teaspoons of hop leaves in a cup and fill with boiling water. Cover the cup and let stand for fifteen minutes. Drink the tea while it's warm. The tea is bitter. Drink one to three cups between dinner and bedtime as needed.

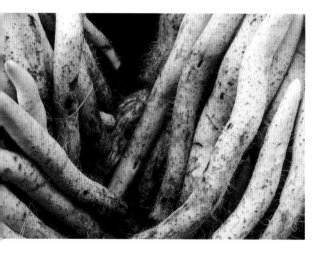

Wild Yam

Wild yam (*Dioscorea villosa*) was used by physicians of the last century to treat spasms of smooth muscle that often accompany gallbladder attacks or painful menstruation. Wild yam contains diosgenin, a steroid constituent with anti-inflammatory properties.

Directions: Place one ounce of wild yam root in a one-quart canning jar. Add a few slices of fresh ginger root. Fill the jar with boiling water, put the lid on tightly, and let the mixture stand until it reaches room temperature. Drink three cups each day for three, then take a break for seven to ten days.

Copper Bracelets

The recommendation for arthritis patients to wear copper bracelets is common throughout European and American folk literature. Copper is a nutrient that may play a role in modifying arthritis. The nutrient takes part in key antioxidant systems that help prevent inflammation and is also necessary for the formation of connective tissue. The normal daily requirement of copper for an adult is 1.5 to 3 milligrams, but that requirement may be higher in patients with rheumatoid arthritis (but not osteoarthritis.)

Directions: Wear a copper bracelet around your wrist or ankle—the more surface area the bracelet covers, the better. (It is unlikely to absorb too much copper. Copper toxicity occurs after ingesting about 60 milligrams of copper, an amount that is many times more than what is found in copper jewelry.)

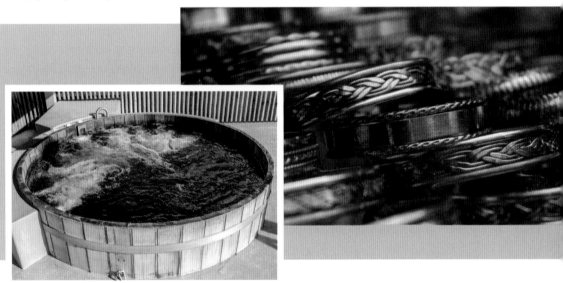

Hydrotherapy

Water treatments for arthritis, which have become popular throughout the United States in the last century, invariably involve heat. Hot water or steam increases the circulation, which in turn can reduce local inflammation and swelling.

Directions: Try one of the following treatments: Take a steam bath in a sauna. Soak in a hot tub, or, if there is one in your area, a hot spring. You can also try placing hot towels on the affected area.

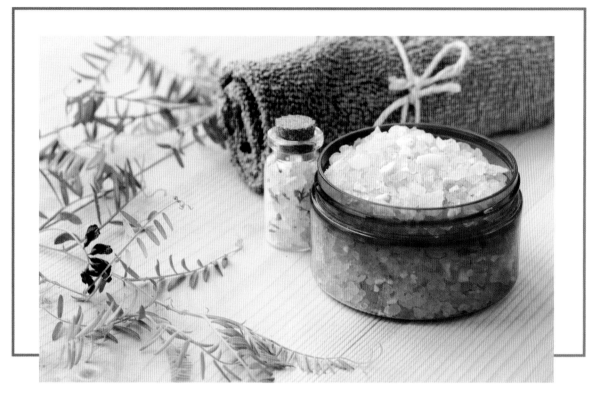

Epsom Salts

In the town of Epsom, England, in 1618, a substance called magnesium sulfate was found in abundance in spring water. The colonists brought the substance, named Epsom salts, to this country. Magnesium has both anti-inflammatory and antiarthritic properties and it can be absorbed through the skin. Magnesium is one of the most important of the essential minerals in the body, and it is commonly deficient in the American diet. A New England remedy for arthritis is a hot bath of Epsom salts. The heat of the bath can increase circulation and reduce the swelling and pain of arthritis.

Directions: *Fill a bathtub with water as hot as you can stand. Add two cups of Epsom salts. Bathe for thirty minutes, adding hot water as necessary to keep the temperature warm. Do this daily as often as you'd like. (If you are pregnant or have cardiovascular disease, however, consult your doctor before taking very hot baths.)*

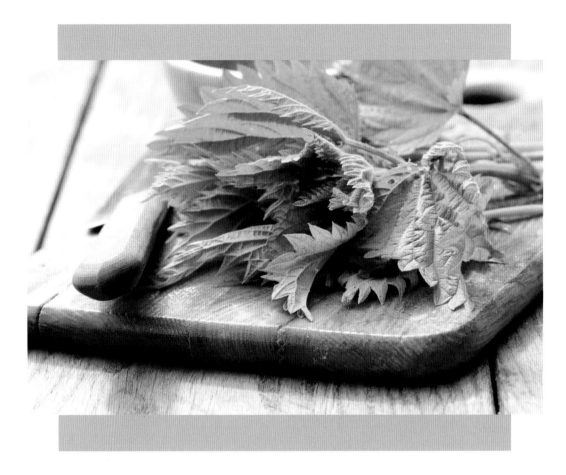

Stinging Nettle

A Romani remedy for arthritis is to drink the juice of nettle leaves. Stinging nettle is an official remedy for rheumatism in Germany. In botanical medicine classes at the National University of Natural Medicine in the United States, it is taught that stinging nettle is the most important herb to consider for treating early-onset arthritis. A 1996 laboratory analysis of nettle juice showed an anti-inflammatory effect similar to that of steroid drugs.

Directions: Purchase nettle leaf juice in a health food store and take as directed on the package. If you know how to identify and harvest nettles, collect your own (they must be harvested before they flower), and juice them in a juicer. Take one tablespoon of nettle juice three times a day. You can freeze the juice for later use. You can also make tea out of dried leaves. Place one ounce of dried nettle in one quart of water. Bring to a boil and then simmer for thirty minutes. Drink three cups a day for as long as you'd like.

Asthma

Asthma affects millions of Americans and claims thousands of lives a year. It is the most common chronic disease among children, affecting one in five. Because it may be a life-threatening condition, any individual with asthma should be under the care of a physician.

Asthma is a respiratory disorder marked by unpredictable periods of acute breathlessness and wheezing. Asthma attacks can last from less than an hour to a week or more and can strike frequently or only every few years. Attacks may be mild or severe and can occur at any time, even during sleep.

The difficult breathing occurs when the small respiratory tubes called bronchioles constrict or become clogged with mucus or when the membranes lining the bronchioles become swollen. When this happens, stale air cannot be fully exhaled but stays trapped in the lungs, so that less fresh air can be inhaled.

Asthma attacks can result from oversensitivity of the bronchial system to a variety of outside substances or conditions. About half of all asthma attacks are triggered by allergies to such substances as dust, smoke,

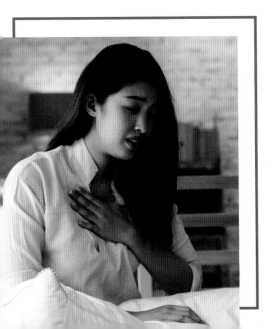

pollen, feathers, pet hair, insects, mold spores, and a variety of foods and drugs. The allergic trigger cannot always be identified, and sometimes food allergens complicate the picture. An individual who is allergic to a specific food may experience "allergic overload" when consuming it and then overreact to a simple pollen or other airborne allergen that normally would not cause a serious problem. Attacks not related to allergies can be set off by strenuous exercise, breathing cold air, stress, and infections of the respiratory tract.

Modern physicians treat asthma with drugs delivered by inhalers, including, in serious cases, steroid drugs. Recent research has demonstrated that prolonged use of inhaled steroids can cause severe side effects similar to those experienced by users of oral steroids, however. Inhaled steroids nevertheless remain an essential and sometimes life-saving part of treatment for severe asthma.

Why does the body overreact to a simple allergen? One possible explanation is a deficiency of the body's natural anti-inflammatory prostaglandins, substances naturally derived from the fats of cold-water fish and wild game. The decline of these foods in the modern diet may be contributing to the increased incidence of asthma. The body can make these substances from certain vegetable oils, but the process is much more complex and can be inhibited by deficiencies of magnesium, zinc, vitamin B6 or vitamin C—all common deficiencies in the modern American diet. Science has linked each of these deficiencies—as well as the reduced consumption of cold-water fish—to asthma, but the evidence is not strong enough to implicate a single deficiency in all cases.

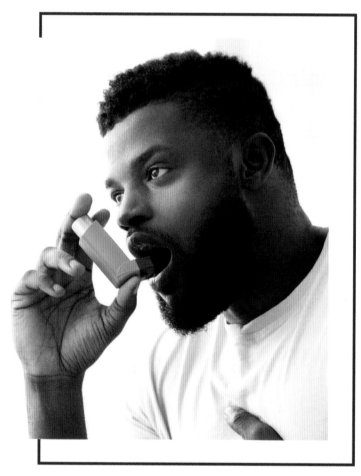

If you suffer from asthma, you might want to consider the natural remedies found here. After all, these remedies have helped the many generations before us breathe a little easier.

remedies for asthma

Mormon Tea

Mormon tea, the common name for a variety of plants in the *Ephedra* genus, has long been used as a decongestant for allergies in western American natural medicines.

The medicinal constituents involved are ephedrine and pseudoephedrine, which also appear in over-the-counter allergy medicines. The American ephedra species do not contain reliable amounts of these constituents. *Ma huang* and ephedrine-containing drug combinations have been responsible for a number of deaths in the United States in recent years, but generally not when taken as allergy medications. Weight-loss formulas and pep pills sometimes contain *ma huang* or ephedrine. In this form they are consumed in much larger amounts than in allergy medications and present a greater risk of side effects. Ephedra is contraindicated in heart disease, hypertension, thyroid conditions, prostate disease, anxiety, pregnancy, and concurrent use of pharmaceutical drugs, except with approval of your physician. Mormon tea itself is not usually available in herb or health food stores, but *ma huang* often is.

Directions: Cover one teaspoon of Chinese ephedra with one cup of boiling water. Let steep for ten minutes. Drink the full cup when suffering an acute asthma attack. Prepare the tea ahead of time and keep it in a sealed container in the refrigerator.

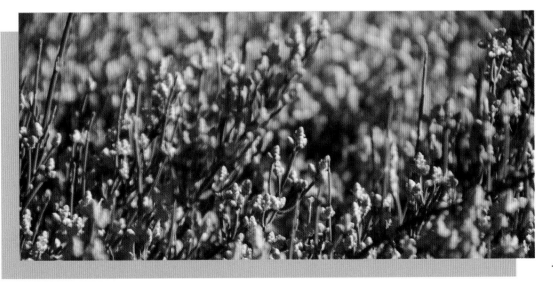

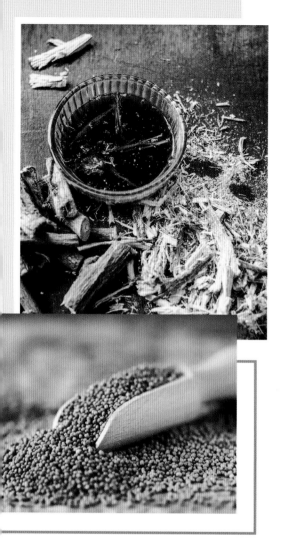

Licorice

Licorice root has long been used to treat coughs and bronchial problems in many cultures throughout the world. It has expectorant properties and also contains anti-inflammatory constituents similar to steroids, although much weaker. Licorice is not so effective in treating an acute asthma attack, but daily use over a long period of time may reduce the body's tendency to overreact to allergens

Directions: Cut one ounce of licorice root into slices, cover with one quart of boiling water, and steep for twenty-four hours. Strain and drink one or two cups a day. Licorice can cause high blood pressure and salt imbalances if taken for long periods. Don't take the above doses if you already have high blood pressure, and don't continue to take the herb in any case for longer than six weeks. (Note: real licorice is not a common ingredient in United States candy. Instead, anise oil is substituted.)

Mustard Seed

An old New England remedy calls for one teaspoon of mustard seed (*Brassica* spp.), taken morning and evening, in the form of a tea or soup. Mustard contains irritating and expectorant sulfur-containing compounds. Like garlic, it can induce vomiting in larger doses and was used for this purpose by the Eclectic physicians of the late 19th and early 20th centuries in cases of narcotic poisoning.

Directions: Crush and moisten the seeds well in order to release the constituents. Let the freshly crushed mustard seeds sit in a warm soup or tea for ten to fifteen minutes before drinking. Take two to three times a day.

Garlic

Garlic (*Allium sativum*) has long been used to treat bronchial problems in many cultures. Like many of the other herbs used to treat asthma, garlic acts as an expectorant in low doses and an emetic in higher doses, especially if taken on an empty stomach.

Directions: Take two cloves of garlic and crush well or blend in a blender. Mix in two cups of hot water. Add a pinch of salt. Drink one cup rapidly. (Though this remedy may induce vomiting, it may also abort the asthma attack.) Then drink a second cup, which will usually stay down better than the first. Also, you can try simmering the garlic in water for twenty minutes. (This destroys some of the irritating substances that cause nausea.) This treatment came from the 12th century German mystic Hildegard von Bingen.

Honey

Honey has been used in traditional Chinese medicine for more than two thousand years. It is used to treat conditions ranging from asthma, cough, and chronic bronchitis to stomachache, constipation, chronic sinus congestion, canker sores, and burns. To cure a cough, a simple remedy from China recommends drinking a tea consisting of hot water and a tablespoon of honey. (This treatment probably isn't strong enough to treat an asthma attack, but it might help thin mucus and prevent congestion.)

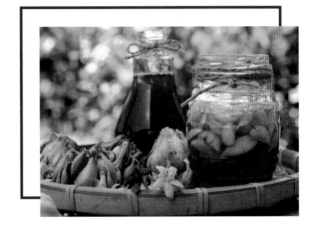

Garlic & Honey

Some syrups combine the healthy benefits of both garlic and honey. Such syrups appear in the traditions of both New England and the Southwest.

Directions: Place eight ounces of peeled and sliced garlic in one pint of boiling water. Let soak for ten to twelve hours, keeping the water warm, but not boiling. Strain and add two pounds of honey. Take one teaspoon of the mixture when you're congested.

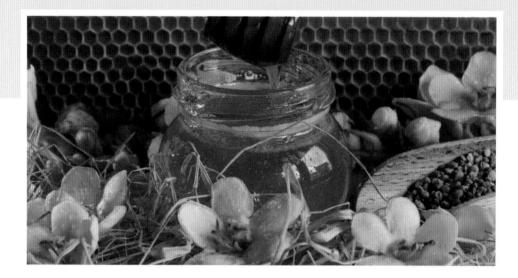

Mullein & Honey

You can use the mullein plant to make an asthma syrup, too. Mullein *(Verbascum thapsus)* came from Europe to North America with the European colonists and is now naturalized throughout the United States and Canada. Its use as a cough medicine was quickly adopted by various Indian tribes. The Penobscot, Potawatomi, and Iroquois tribes used mullein specifically to treat asthma. It was an official medicine in the *United States Pharmacopoeia* from 1888 to 1936.

Directions: *Place ½ pound of mullein leaves in a one-quart jar. Fill the jar with boiling water and let cool to room temperature. Strain. Add honey to the tea until it is the consistency of syrup. Take one tablespoon of the syrup when suffering an asthma attack.*

Nettle & Honey

This home remedy comes from German immigrants who settled in the New York area. Nettle juice *(Urtica dioica, Urtica urens)* and nettle syrups may still be purchased in Germany today. American physicians of the 19th and early 20th centuries also used nettle to treat some types of allergic conditions. Nettle is an unusually mineral-rich plant. An ounce of the dried herb contains more than two-thirds of the minimum daily requirement of magnesium, which is a frequently deficient mineral in asthma patients.

Directions: *Take ½ pint of nettle juice, boil it, remove the scum from the pot, and mix the remaining juice with an equal part of honey. Take one tablespoonful in the morning and evening.*

Daisy Blossoms

White daisy blossoms (*Chrysanthemum leucanthemum*) were an early traditional asthma remedy in the eastern United States. By the turn of the 20th century, this plant had become a standard medical treatment of the Eclectic physicians.

Directions: Take four ounces of white daisy blossoms and crush them well. Pour one pint of boiling water over them. Steep for one hour and strain. Take three tablespoons two to three times a day.

Elder Flower Pillow

Another remedy from the eastern states of the last century is to sleep on a pillow stuffed with dried elder leaves or flowers (*Sambucus* spp.). As you sleep, you'll inhale the plant's aromatic oils and breathe a little easier.

Directions: Take four ounces of dried elder leaves or flowers and place inside a pillow. (Be careful of allergic reactions to the flower's pollen.)

Foot Bath & Tea

A Seventh Day Adventist treatment for asthma is to induce sweating by putting the feet in warm water and drinking a tea made of catnip (*Napeta cataria*) or pennyroyal (*Hedeoma pulegioides*). Catnip and pennyroyal are both diaphoretics—they bring circulation to the skin and produce sweating. Don't use this treatment during pregnancy, however; both these herbs promote menstruation.

Directions: Fill a bathtub or a smaller tub with hot water. Put the feet in the water while drinking the hot tea. (This treatment is contraindicated in diabetics, however, because the feet might be burned.)

To make the tea, place one ounce of catnip or pennyroyal leaves in a one-quart jar and cover with boiling water. Cover the jar tightly and let steep for ten to fifteen minutes. Strain and drink.

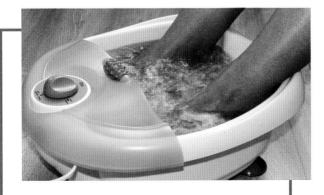

Eggshells & Molasses

An early 18th century asthma treatment in the eastern United States was to mix roasted eggshells with blackstrap molasses. This mixture makes an effective mineral supplement. The eggshells are almost pure calcium carbonate, and molasses is one of the most mineral-rich foods on earth. The dose of molasses below contains a significant portion of the recommended dietary allowance of magnesium, and this amount has been found in some scientific studies to be an effective treatment for asthma. (The treatment is remarkably similar to a traditional Mongolian remedy for leg cramps due to calcium deficiency, where black pepper berries are mixed with eggshells, which are roasted until brown and then crushed into powder.)

Directions: *Roast three eggshells until brown. Crush into a powder. Mix with half of a pint of molasses. The dose is one tablespoonful three times a day for as long as desired.*

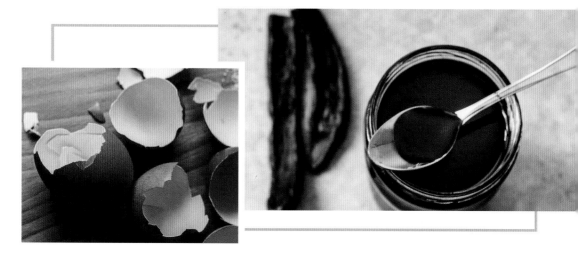

Herbal Formula

A tea formula from the last century combines licorice root *(Glycyrrhiza glabra)*, mullein leaves *(Verbascum thapsus)*, horehound leaves *(Marrubium vulgare)*, lungwort *(Pulmonaria officinalis)*, and sage *(Salvia officinalis)*. All these herbs have subsequently been used in North American, British, and German herbal medicine, and licorice, mullein, horehound, and sage have all been listed as official medicines in the *United States Pharmacopoeia.*

Directions: *Place ½ ounce of each of the herbs in one quart of water. Boil for twenty minutes. Strain when cool. Drink five ounces at bedtime.*

Botanical Beauty

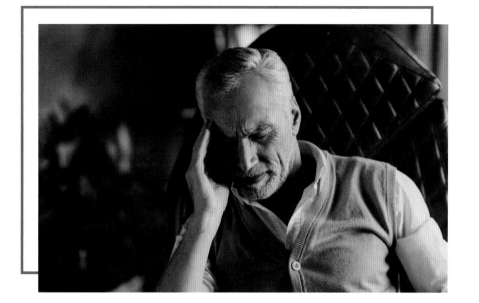

A headache is a symptom of disease, and not a disease in itself. Rarely is a headache the symptom of a serious illness—most headaches are caused by minor conditions, such as muscle tension in the neck and around the skull or inflammation of blood vessels in the brain.

There are three basic types of headaches. The vascular headache occurs when blood vessels in the head enlarge and press on nerves, causing pain. The most common vascular headache is the migraine. The second type of headache is the muscle contraction headache, which results when the muscles of the face, neck, or scalp contract and tighten. A tension headache is an example of a muscle contraction headache. The third kind of headache is the inflammatory headache. Such a headache is the result of pressure within the head. The causes range from relatively minor conditions, such as sinusitis, to more serious problems, such as brain tumors.

Headaches are most often treated with aspirin and nonsteroidal anti-inflammatory drugs (NSAIDs) such as ibuprofen or acetaminophen. Treatment of a migraine already in progress usually consists of a drug therapy program chosen from a variety of painkillers, sedatives, and special drugs and remedies, including vasoconstricting drugs and caffeine. Tension headaches can be treated by eliminating the tension or correcting the physical problem that is causing the headaches. This can sometimes be done through physical manipulation of the spine or skull by a chiropractic or osteopathic physician.

The herbal remedies for headaches, which are still used today by alternative physicians in the United States and by some conventional doctors in Europe, fall into four categories: pain-relievers, anti-inflammatories, sedatives, and digestive herbs. The pain-relieving and anti-inflammatory herbs may relieve most types of headaches. The sedatives work well for relieving tension headaches. The digestive herbs and laxatives are most useful for treating headaches that accompany digestive sluggishness or constipation.

remedies for headaches

Most people find that their headaches respond best to a cold compress, but you can use a warm or hot compress—or alternate the two—for the result that works best. You can also place a second compress at the back of the neck. When you do not have time for compresses, dab a small drop of lavender, eucalyptus, or peppermint oil on each temple. For some people, a hot bath only makes their head pound more. However, if bathing does ease your pain, add a few drops of relaxing lavender or chamomile to your bath water.

Migraine headaches can be especially painful. Raising the temperature of the hands a few degrees by soaking them in warm water seems to short-circuit a vascular headache such as a migraine by regulating circulation. Adding a couple drops of essential oil to the water increases the effect. Migraines often respond best to a blend of ginger and lavender.

Cluster headaches can also be quite severe and require special treatment. In addition to the headache compress, try a cream made from capsaicin, the active compound in cayenne peppers. Spread it on your forehead, temples, or any other area where you experience pain, but not too close to the eyes. Capsaicin blocks a neurotransmitter called substance P (which stands for pain), stopping pain impulses from registering in the brain. The cream works best as a preventative, keeping the headache from forming in the first place.

Rosemary-Sage Tea

A natural remedy for treating headache pain is to drink a tea of rosemary (*Rosmarinus officinalis*) and sage (*Salvia officinalis*). Rosemary has been a popular medicine in Europe for treating pain at least since the time of the ancient Greeks.

Today, rosemary is used to soothe headaches in the traditional medicine of China. The German government has approved the use of rosemary for pain. There, rosemary is often used externally, in preparations such as salves and baths. It is a common folk use to apply rosemary to the temples in the form of a poultice to relieve headache pain.

Sage is not often used in natural medicine as a pain reliever, but it has an important chemical constituent in common with rosemary—rosmarinic acid. In addition, the combination of rosemary and sage contains more than twenty anti-inflammatory constituents, although some of these exist only in minute amounts. Seek medical attention for any headache that lasts longer than three days. Do not ingest rosemary in any amount exceeding those usually found in foods because of the herb's reputed abortifacient and emmenagogue effects.

Directions: Place one teaspoon of crushed rosemary leaves and one teaspoon of crushed sage leaves in a cup. Fill with boiling water. Cover well to prevent the escape of volatile substances. Let steep until the tea reaches room temperature. Take ½-cup doses two or three times a day for two or three days. You don't have to mix rosemary and sage to find pain relief. You can also try drinking either rosemary or sage teas separately.

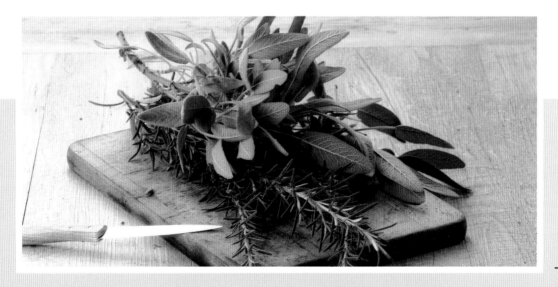

American Pennyroyal

Pennyroyal tea (*Hedeoma pulegioides*) is a headache remedy from the Onondaga tribe. In European medicine, a European species of pennyroyal (*Mentha pulegioides L.*) is used for pain relief. In fact, the 17th century British herbalist John Gerard wrote of pennyroyal: "A Garland of Pennie Royall made and worn about the head is of great force against swimming in the head, and the paines and giddiness thereof." The use of pennyroyal for treating headaches persists today in the natural medicine of Appalachia and Indiana. Pennyroyal contains significant amounts of the anti-inflammatory substance diosmin.

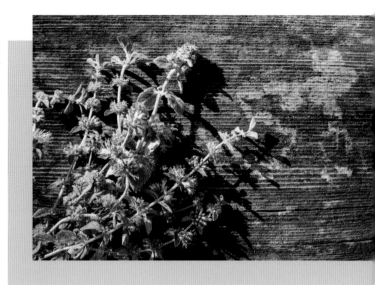

Directions: Place one teaspoon of dried pennyroyal leaves in a cup and fill with boiling water. Cover well to avoid the loss of volatile constituents. Let steep. Take ½-cup doses as desired, up to four times a day.

Coffee or Tea

Coffee or tea is recommended as a headache cure in several traditions. Caffeine is the medicinal constituent responsible for the benefits. Caffeine is also used in conventional medicine to treat migraine headaches. It works by constricting the vessels of the brain, which are sometimes dilated during a headache attack. Tea is recommended in New England, and strong black coffee in Appalachia. Black coffee is a famous cure throughout Europe and North America for the type of headache that accompanies hangover.

Directions: Make a pot of strong black coffee or tea and drink two cups to relieve an acute headache.

Laxatives

Clarence Meyer suggests taking low doses of laxatives to cure a headache. This remedy is best used on headaches that accompany constipation. The habitual use of laxatives is not recommended, however.

Directions: Place ¼ teaspoon of senna leaves in a cup. Add ¼ teaspoon of sage leaves and ¼ teaspoon of powdered ginger. Fill the cup with boiling water. Let steep until cool. Drink a cup every four hours. Do not exceed three doses in a day. Do not repeat the treatment for a second day. If the constipation and headache persist, see a physician. Do not use laxatives during pregnancy.

Mints

The mints—peppermint *(Mentha piperita)* and spearmint *(mentha spicata)*—are used as headache remedies in the medicine of the particular regions where they grow. American Indians of both eastern and western North America, including the Cherokee, Iroquois, Gosuite, and Paiute tribes, used these mints as headache remedies. Some tribes crushed the plant and inhaled the fumes; others placed the plant on the forehead or temples.

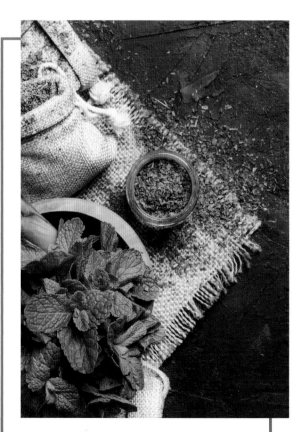

Today, the mints contain about the same levels of the anti-inflammatory rosmarinic acid as do rosemary and sage.

Directions: Place one ounce of dried mint leaves in a one-quart jar and fill with boiling water. Cover tightly to prevent the escape of the aromatic constituents. The dose is ½ cup of tea, two to four times a day.

Wormwood

Plants of the Artemisia genus *(Artemisia spp.)* have been used as pain remedies by at least twenty-two Native American tribes throughout North America. Some tribes received the pain-relieving properties of the plants by burning them and inhaling their smoke and aromatic oils. To treat a headache, others made tea from the leaves and used them as a wash on the forehead and temples. The use of the *Artemisia* species is recorded today in the natural medicine of northern New Mexico. Excessive use in large amounts can lead to brain damage, however.

The active constituents of plants in the *Artemisia* species include bitter digestive stimulants and anti-inflammatory volatile oils such as azulenes. These constituents are also present in yarrow and chamomile.

Directions: Place one teaspoon of wormwood leaves in a cup of water and fill with boiling water. Cover well. Let cool to room temperature. Take ½-cup doses every three hours for up to three days.

migraine headache hand soak

-5 drops lavender oil
-5 drops ginger oil
-1 quart hot water, about 100 degrees Fahrenheit

Directions: Add essential oils to the hot water, and soak hands for at least three minutes. This therapy can be done repeatedly.

restful headache pillow

-12 drops lavender oil   -1 cup flax seeds
-12 drops marjoram oil   -Small piece of silk cloth

Directions: *Add essential oils to flax seeds (found at any natural food store) in a glass jar and let them sit for a week until the oils are absorbed. Fold and stitch the cloth (an old scarf works fine) into a bag and add the scented flax seeds. Sew up the opening. Lie down, and lay this "pillow" over your eyes when you feel a headache coming on. Store the pillow in a glass jar to preserve the scent. If the scent starts to dissipate, you can add more essential oil directly through the cloth as needed.*

headache-be-gone compress

-5 drops lavender or eucalyptus oil
-1 cup cold water

Directions: *Add essential oil to water, and swish a soft cloth in it. Wring out the cloth, lie down, and close your eyes. Place the cloth over your forehead and eyes. Use throughout the day, as often as you can.*

At some point in our lives, between one third and one half of all Americans have a serious bout of chronic insomnia, which is the inability to sleep the desired amount at least three nights a week for a month or more. Insomnia may mean difficulty falling asleep, waking up periodically during the night, or waking up too early. Length of sleep is not a measure of insomnia, because different people require different amounts. So, if disturbed sleep leaves you feeling fatigued and not up to par the next day, you may be suffering from insomnia, even if you slept for eight hours. Brief spells of insomnia may accompany worry, stress, changes in job shifts, or other temporary life situations. Habitual coffee drinking, even if only a few cups a day, may also cause or contribute to insomnia. Chronic insomnia may accompany such conditions as depression; chronic pain; or withdrawal from nicotine, alcohol, drugs, or sleep medications; or life passages such as menopause. Because some of these conditions become more prevalent as we age, insomnia is common among the elderly.

Insomnia can be the first sign of nutritional deficiencies, appearing before more serious diseases arise. It may indicate a deficiency of calcium, magnesium, or potassium,

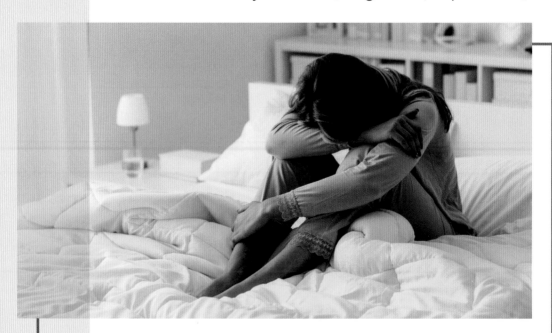

all of which are common deficiencies in the American diet. Deficiencies of the B-vitamins or of vitamin E may also cause insomnia.

Chronic stress can also lead to insomnia. Our body possesses hormonal mechanisms to respond to brief periods of stress throughout the day. At night, our body is given a break from these mechanisms to recuperate. When the body adapts to persistent stress, however, we end up physically prepared to run from a bear, even at bedtime, when we should be resting. Many of the natural remedies in this section help send cues to the brain, body, and glandular system that we are safe and that it is now time to relax and recuperate in order to meet the challenges and stresses of tomorrow.

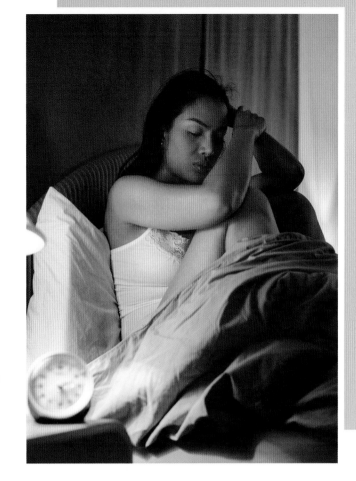

Conventional medical treatment for chronic insomnia includes drugs in the benzodiazepine class, such as Valium and Xanax. These drugs may be appropriate to induce sleep during a brief crisis, but withdrawal from them may worsen the insomnia or induce anxiety, and use for as little as six weeks may cause addiction. These drugs, as well as over-the-counter sleep medications, can also disrupt patterns of sleep, interfering with the deepest stage of sleep known as deep delta-wave sleep. During this part of sleep, the body normally recovers from stress, rebuilds its immune system, and repairs tissues. Chronic drug use can result in a constant feeling of fatigue, however. Before you turn to prescription or over-the-counter medications, you may want to try one of the remedies below for a healthier, more natural snooze.

remedies for insomnia

Pine, Juniper, & Sage

A very common aromatherapy technique to induce sleep uses the scents of pine (*Pinus* spp.), juniper (*Juniperus* spp.), or sage (*Artemesia* spp., *Salvia* spp.). The remedy requires burning and then inhaling the fresh or dried needles or leaves of the herbs. Also, you can inhale the scent by pouring a tea made from the dried plant over hot rocks.

Directions: You can adapt this technique for household use by burning the dried needles or leaves like incense. Take some dried needles or leaves of pine, juniper, or sage, light them with a match, blow the flame out, and put the smoking embers in an ashtray. Inhale the fragrance as it fills the room.

Massage

Scientific research shows that massage can induce relaxation and ease stress.

Directions: Massage the patient gently, with the strokes always moving in the direction of the heart.

Herbal Baths

When you bathe with herbs, your skin absorbs their essential oils. You can add relaxing herbs to any of the baths previously described. Avoid using oils such as peppermint, clove, and cinnamon, however. These hot oils can burn sensitive skin.

Directions: Place one ounce of valerian, hop, chamomile, or lavender in a pot and cover with a quart of boiling water. Strain and add the water to the bath. Another approach is to add two drops of essential oil to the tub water. Remember that herbal oils are highly concentrated, so a little goes a long way. Enjoy an herbal bath right before bedtime.

Botanical Beauty

Dill Seeds

A natural remedy from China is to wash the head in a tea of dill seeds (*Anethum graveoveolens*) so you'll inhale the fumes of the tea. Dill contains a number of sedative constituents in its volatile oil, which may

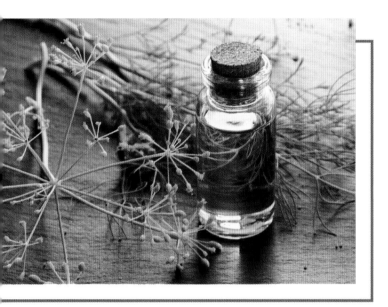

explain the value of the plant for insomnia. Dill itself has not been tested by scientists for these purposes.

Directions: Put ten drops of essential oil of dill in one ounce of another oil, such as almond oil. Apply the mixture to a cloth, and keep it near your nose while you sleep. No direct application to the head is necessary.

The Hop Pillow

A widespread cure for insomnia is the hop pillow. Hop (*Humulus lupulus*) has been used for centuries as a mild sedative. Hop was listed as an official medicine in the *United States Pharmacopoeia* from 1820 to 1926.

Directions: Cut two eight-by-eleven-inch squares of muslin fabric. Place one muslin square on top of the other and pin together around the edges. Sew ½-inch seams along the two long sides and one short side of the fabric, leaving the second short side open. Turn the seams to the inside. Take four ounces of hop, the fresher the better. Sprinkle it with a small amount of alcohol to bring out the active principle, but not enough to make it soggy. Add the herb to the muslin pillow case. Spread the herbs evenly within the pillow. Turn the raw edges under and pin the opening shut to enclose the content of the pillow securely.

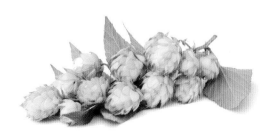

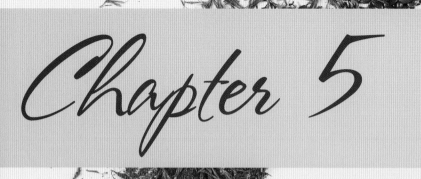

Chapter 5

SECRET FIXES FOR EYES, TEETH, AND MORE

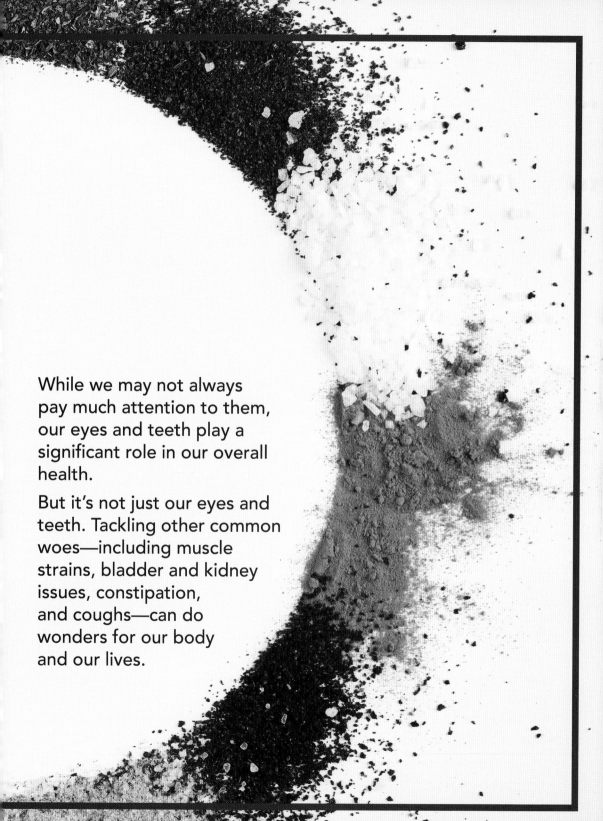

While we may not always pay much attention to them, our eyes and teeth play a significant role in our overall health.

But it's not just our eyes and teeth. Tackling other common woes—including muscle strains, bladder and kidney issues, constipation, and coughs—can do wonders for our body and our lives.

Eyes

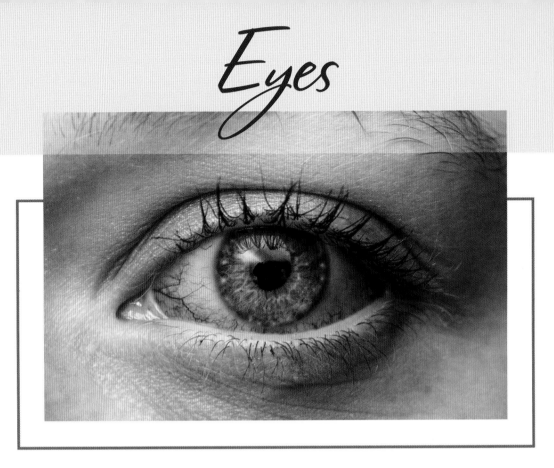

Conjunctivitis, or pinkeye, is an inflammation of the conjunctiva. The conjunctiva is a delicate membrane that lines the inner surface of the eyelid and covers the exposed surface of the eye. Most cases of conjunctivitis result from disease-causing microorganisms such as bacteria, fungi, and viruses. Allergies, chemicals, dust, smoke, and foreign objects that irritate the conjunctiva may also lead to conjunctivitis. (Occasionally a sexually transmitted disease can cause pinkeye if the eyes are rubbed after touching infected organs. Herpes simplex keratitis is a viral infection of the cornea of the eye that can result in blindness if not treated.)

Most cases of conjunctivitis in North America are caused by viruses. In Asia and the Mediterranean region, however, eye infections are commonly caused by the organism Chlamydia trachomatis. Known as trachoma, this persistent infection can cause scarring and excessive drying of the membranes around the eyes and lead to blindness.

Conventional treatment depends upon the cause and resulting symptoms of the conjunctivitis. If the inflammation is environmentally caused, simply removing the irritant may be sufficient to eliminate the condition. For more difficult cases, a physician may prescribe antibiotics, steroids, or combination eye drops to be used several times a day as directed.

A most important fact about conjunctivitis is that its infectious form is highly contagious. Individuals with infective conjunctivitis should not share handkerchiefs, towels, or washcloths. You should be careful to avoid touching the unaffected eye after touching or rubbing the infected eye because it can easily become infected as well.

The most common natural remedies for the eyes focus on relieving infected, sore, or tired eyes as well as removing irritating objects. (Of course, caution should be used when removing a foreign object from the eye. Sometimes even small objects can tear the surface of the eyeball or cornea, and infection can result. Use common sense.) The natural treatments for treating conjunctivitis commonly employ drying substances, which give tone to swollen membranes around the eyes. Some of the herbs recommended also have antibacterial, antiviral, and anti-inflammatory properties.

Any persistent eye irritation or infection requires a medical checkup.

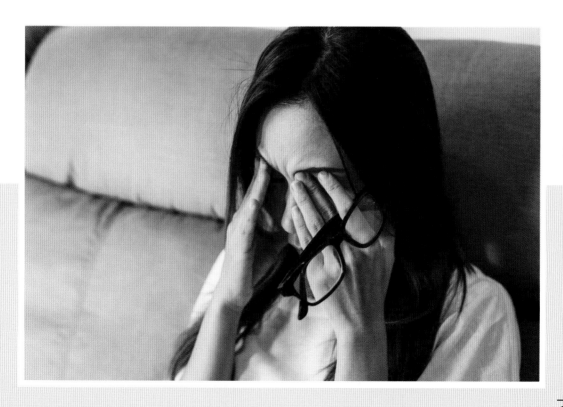

remedies for eye issues

Rose

Rose petals have a strong astringent action, toning up swollen and inflamed mucous membranes. The rose oil in the leaves contains fifteen bactericidal, nine antiviral, and seven anti-inflammatory constituents.

Directions: Obtain rose petals from wild or garden-cultivated roses that are free of pesticides and chemicals. (Most commercial roses are sprayed with a variety of chemicals.) Place a handful of petals in a jar and add one pint of boiling water. Cover well to retain the aromatic oils, and let stand until the water reaches room temperature. Apply to the eyes with a clean cloth.

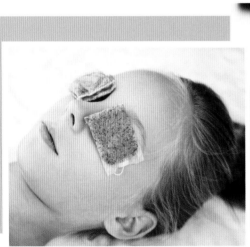
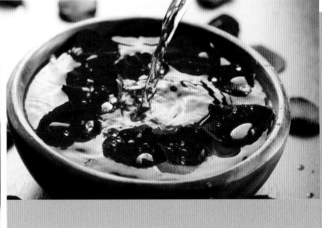

Tea

Tea and tea leaves are used to treat all types of eye irritations and infections, including runny eyes, conjunctivitis, particles in the eye, swollen eyelids, sticky eyelids, and eyes red from a hangover.

Tea is a virtual pharmacy of chemical constituents: The leaves contain thirty-four antibacterial substances, sixteen antiviral substances, and twenty-four anti-inflammatory constituents. Tea leaves also have a strong astringent action, which soothes inflamed membranes.

Directions: Make tea using black or green tea bags or by adding one teaspoon of tea leaves to one cup of boiling water. Apply a tea-soaked cloth or a used tea bag, to the eyes. Keep in place for ten to fifteen minutes. Repeat as desired.

Botanical Beauty

Witch Hazel

Witch hazel is a tree native to North America. After colonists learned its importance from Native Americans, its use for healing spread to Europe. The German government, after reviewing scientific evidence, has approved its use for minor inflammation of the skin and mucous membranes. Witch hazel products are available in most drug stores and health food stores.

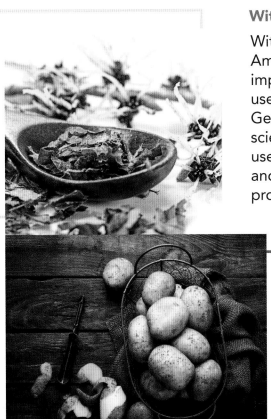

Directions: *Purchase witch hazel leaves at a health food store or herb shop. Do not use commercial alcohol-based preparations—the alcohol will irritate your eyes. Place one teaspoon of the leaves in a cup and fill with boiling water. Cover and let stand until the water reaches room temperature. Moisten a cloth in the tea and apply to shut eyes.*

Potato Poultice

A remedy recorded in Clarence Meyer's *American Folk Medicine* is the potato poultice. Presumably, the starch in the potato acts to soothe the inflammation in the eye. Small amounts of a number of other anti-inflammatory constituents are also present in the potato.

The potato is native to the Andes mountains in South America. Its use as a food spread throughout Europe in the 1700s. It is used today in European natural medicine to soothe painful joints, headaches, and other inflammatory conditions.

Directions: *Remove the skin from a whole, raw potato. Wash the potato and dry well. Grate as fine as possible. Place inside a clean cloth and fold to make a poultice. Place the poultice over the inflamed eye for fifteen minutes.*

Oregon Grape Root

A tea of the roots or leaves of Oregon grape root (*Mahonia* spp., *Berberis aquifolium)* was used as an eyewash by Native Americans of both the mountainous American Southwest and the Pacific Northwest. The use of Oregon grape root for this purpose eventually spread to the settlers in those areas. Oregon grape root contains the alkaloid berberine, which acts as an antibiotic when used topically.

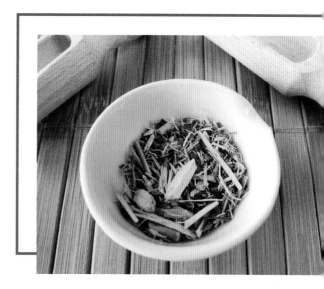

Directions: Place ½ ounce of Oregon grape root in a pot and add one pint of boiling water. Let cool to room temperature. Apply to the eyes with a clean cloth.

Goldenseal

During the second decade of the 19th century, American botanist Constantine Rafinesque traveled among the Native Americans of the Ohio River and Mississippi River valleys, recording their uses of plants. His work resulted in *Medical Flora*, the first scientific book of medical botany in the United States. In his research, Rafinesque discovered that the Indians in the Midwest used goldenseal as a specific treatment for sore, inflamed, or infected eyes. They made an eyewash by boiling the root in water. This and other uses for goldenseal were quickly adopted by the European settlers in the eastern United States.

Part of goldenseal's medicinal action on the eyes is due to its constituents hydrastine and berberine. Like several other remedies in this section, it also has an astringent effect on swollen mucous membranes. Treating eye infections is one of the few legitimate medical uses for goldenseal.

Because goldenseal is no longer readily available, other berberine-containing herbs, including Oregon grape root, are less expensive, yet still effective substitutes.

Directions: Boil a handful of goldenseal root in one quart of water for twenty minutes. Let cool to room temperature. Apply to the eyes with a clean cloth.

Botanical Beauty

Chrysanthemum

A Chinese treatment for tired, bloodshot, or sore eyes is a tea of dried chrysanthemum flowers.

Chrysanthemum (*Chrysanthemum indicum flos.*) is a popular beverage that can be found throughout the United States.

Chinese and Japanese researchers have found constituents in chrysanthemum tea that inhibit *Staphylococcus* bacteria, a common cause of eye infection in some parts of the world. Chrysanthemum is also effective against a wide variety of other bacteria and viruses.

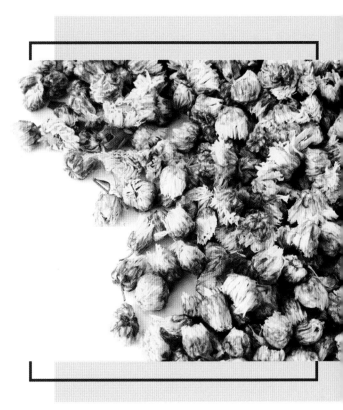

Directions: *Obtain chrysanthemum flowers from a health food store, herb shop, or market. Purchase the whole dried flowers instead of a prepared tea. Place a large handful of the flowers in a pot and add one quart of boiling water. Cover and steep for ten minutes. Strain, setting aside the still-warm flowers. Drink a cup of the tea. Wrap the flowers in a clean cloth, and, while lying down, apply to the eyes until the flowers are cool.*

Eye Bath

Eye baths can remove objects from the eyes.

Directions: *Use a bowl large enough to completely immerse the face. Fill the bowl with cold water. Open the eyes underwater several times, until the object is washed out. Eye cups are still available in some pharmacies and are very convenient to use.*

Dental problems are perhaps the oldest known conditions to afflict humanity. Prehistoric skulls from 25,000 years ago show signs of tooth decay. Remedies for tooth, mouth, and gum problems have probably existed at least since that time. By 3700 B.C., the Egyptians were using tiny drills to make a hole in the jaw to drain an infected tooth. By 2700 B.C., the Chinese had begun to treat tooth pain with acupuncture. The Greek physician Aesculapius introduced the pulling of diseased teeth in Greece sometime around 1200 B.C. It was the barbers who pulled teeth in 17th century England.

Reliable dental anesthetics only became available in the United States during the 1800s; anesthetics were still not available in some isolated areas of this country as late as the early 1970s, however. Understandably, then, many natural remedies for toothache, mouth pain, and gum disease survive into the present day in spite of more reliable professional dental care.

The best medicine for dental problems is prevention, which means regular cleaning of the teeth. Diet also has a strong impact on dental health, and, unfortunately, our

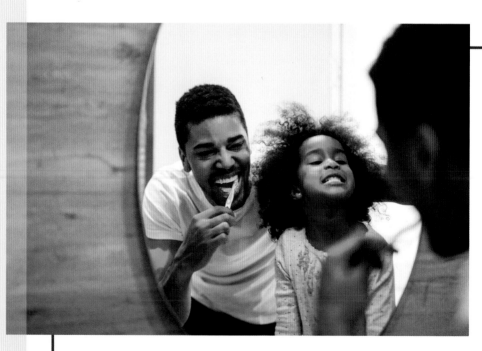

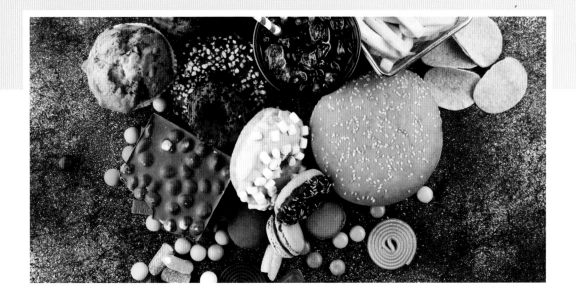

modern processed foods promote tooth decay. During the 1930s, dentist and researcher Weston Price visited more than 20 traditional cultures, including residents of Europe, Africa, North and South America, Australia, and the South Sea Islands. In each place, he examined the teeth of the inhabitants who ate a traditional diet and the teeth of those who ate modern foods, which were just being introduced into their villages at that time. The people eating the traditional diets averaged from one to four percent dental cavities, while those eating the modern foods averaged from twenty to forty percent. The culprits among the foods were sugar and white flour.

The chief risk of unattended dental cavities is a dental abscess—an infection at the roots of the tooth within the jawbone. An abscess can sometimes be "silent" and cause no pain. But it may cause systemic infection and health problems far beyond the site of the infection. An abscess may require removal of the tooth. Sometimes a root canal operation is performed. In that procedure, the nerves and vascular tissue (pulp) within the tooth are removed, a disinfectant is put into the root canal, and the tooth is filled. Teeth can be "saved" in this manner and last for many decades, or even for life.

Most of the remedies in this section are for treating gum disease or sores in the mouth. If you suffer from gum disease, remember to regularly clean your teeth—you also need to floss and go for a periodic cleaning at your dentist's office. The remedies here, including the ones for dental pain, may still come in handy, though.

remedies for a healthy mouth

Clove

Clove *(Eugenia caryophyllata)* has been used as a toothache remedy in Asia since antiquity. Later, it moved along trade routes from Europe to the Mediterranean. By 3 B.C., clove had become a universal natural remedy for dental pain in the Mediterranean. Dentists of the 19th century, in both Europe and North America, also used clove oil to relieve dental pain. Today, dentists use eugenol, a major ingredient in oil of clove, to relieve dental pain and to disinfect dental abscesses. Eugenol also has local anesthetic properties.

Directions: Blend up one teaspoon of clove into a powder in a coffee grinder. Moisten the powder with some olive oil and pack into a cavity or area where a filling has been lost. Alternately, you can purchase clove oil at a pharmacy or health food store. Soak a cotton ball with the oil and place on the gums next to an aching tooth. Be sure to visit your dentist promptly to prevent further tooth decay.

Willow

The bark of various species of the willow tree *(Salix* spp.) have been used to treat mouth and gum infections for hundreds of years. Although willow bark is famous for its aspirin-like constituents, it has antimicrobial constituents as well. The bark is also astringent, which can tone swollen gum tissues.

Directions: Place one ounce of willow bark in one quart of water. Bring to a boil, cover, and simmer on the lowest heat for twenty minutes. Remove from heat and let stand until the water reaches room temperature. Refrigerate and use as a mouthwash up to eight times a day.

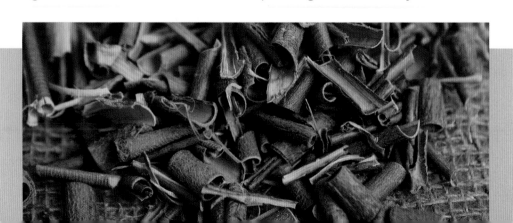

Echinacea

Echinacea was a universal toothache and gum disease remedy among the Native Americans of the Great Plains region. Although it formerly grew in abundance in that area, echinacea is rapidly disappearing in that region due to overharvesting for worldwide medicinal use. Applied topically to skin or gums, echinacea can promote the healing of wounds and ulcers.

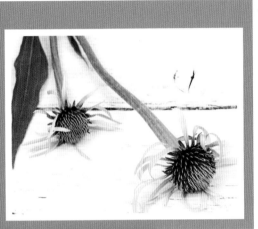

Directions: Obtain a whole or chopped Echinacea angustifolia root at a health food store or herb shop. Grind a small amount in a coffee grinder. Pack the powder like snuff between your cheek and the tooth next to a sore area, or pack the powder directly into a cavity. Be sure to see your dentist at the first opportunity so that tooth decay does not progress.

Yerba Mansa

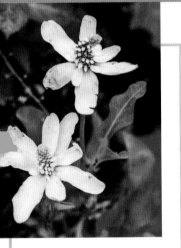

What goldenseal was to the Native Americans of the eastern forests (and echinacea was to the Plains Indians), yerba mansa (*Anemopsis californica*) was to the American Southwest. All three herbs were used as panaceas for a wide variety of illnesses. Spanish settlers learned the uses of yerba mansa from the Maricopa, Pima, Tewa, and Yaqui tribes. (*Yerba mansa* is short for *yerba del indio manso,* or "herb of the tamed Indians.")

Yerba mansa contains the volatile constituents thymol and methyl eugenol, both of which have demonstrated antimicrobial properties. Its other constituents, which are similar to those in goldenseal and myrrh gum, are astringent. Use yerba mansa for treating sores in the mouth.

Directions: Place one ounce of yerba mansa in one quart of water, bring to a boil, and simmer for twenty to thirty minutes. Let stand. Refrigerate. Use as a mouthwash for gum disease or mouth sores as often as eight times a day.

Secret Fixes for Eyes, Teeth, and More

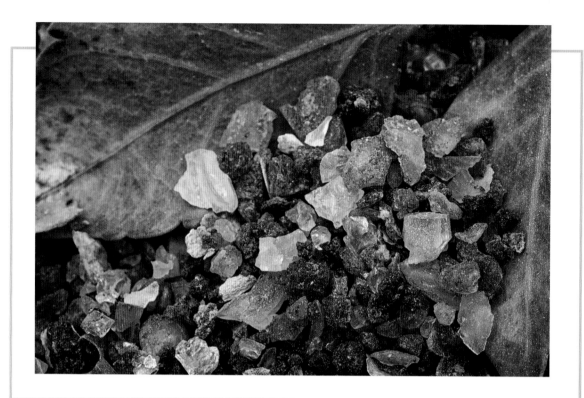

Myrrh Gum

Myrrh gum (*Commiphora myrrha*) has been used to treat mouth problems in the Middle East and North Africa since antiquity. Myrrh gum is astringent and tightens up loose gums. It is also antimicrobial. (The Egyptians used it in their mummification process to prevent the bacterial degradation of the corpse.) The following toothache remedy comes from an 1846 herbal tincture of the Thomsonian tradition.

Directions: *Combine one and a half ounces of myrrh gum and one teaspoon of cayenne pepper in a jar containing a pint of brandy. Cover the jar, and shake it several times a day for a week. Strain and save the brandy. You now have a tincture. To treat a toothache, dip a cotton ball in the tincture and place it on the cavity. Be sure to see a dentist at the first opportunity to prevent further tooth decay.*

To treat swollen and inflamed gums, make a mouthwash by combining a one-ounce shot glass of the tincture with three ounces of water. Rinse the mouth frequently during the day.

Muscle Strains and Sprains

When the body's tissues are injured, the body initiates the process of inflammation to heal them. Blood flow increases to the area, causing redness. Lymph floods the tissues, causing swelling. (The initial flooding of lymph to the area can cause severe pain as the tissues are stretched.) Chemicals that cause pain are secreted to the damaged tissues. The net effect of all this swelling and pain is to immobilize the area to prevent further injury.

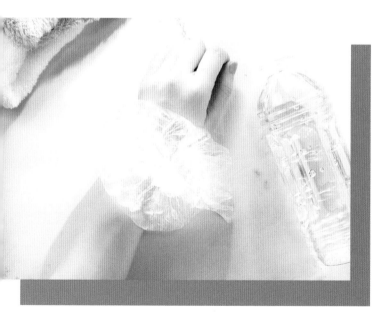

Next, some of the body's white blood cells migrate to the area to clear away damaged tissue. Good circulation is necessary at this stage to bring in the nutrients necessary to build new tissue and carry away the debris of the injury.

You can decrease the pain in the area by reducing the swelling. Soak the affected part in cool water. After the first day, however, it is important to increase circulation to the injured part. To do this, treat the area with hot soaks and massage.

Homeopathic Arnica

One of the most popular homeopathic remedies in the United States health food stores in arnica, which is used for bruises, strains, sprains, and other painful traumas. Homeopathic remedies are highly diluted substances and are a subject of controversy in science because they often contain no traces of the original substance. Clinical trials show that some homeopathic remedies have a medicinal effect, but conventional scientists cannot explain why they work. Homeopathic arnica supposedly will relieve traumatic pain that is accompanied by bruising and has been used this way by homeopaths for several centuries.

Chinese "Hit" Medicine

One branch of traditional Chinese herbal medicine, called "hit medicine," deals with the treatment of traumatic injuries. In any North American Asian market that sells herbal medicines, you can find these internal and external medicines for strains, sprains, and bruises. Liniments and plasters that stick to your skin, and other formulas, are also available.

Directions: Some formulas to look for are Yunnan Pi Yao, an internal formula shown in clinical trials to reduce internal bleeding and bruising; White Flower Analgesic Balm, an external liniment; and Po Sum On medicated oil, which is also for external use.

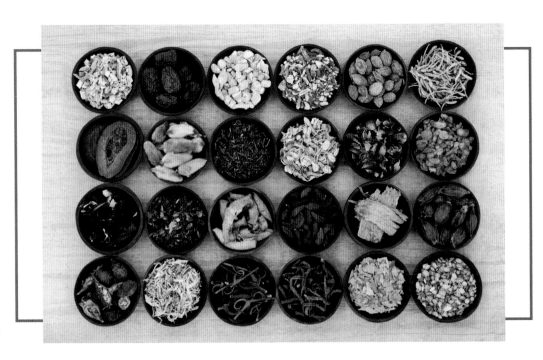

Cayenne Peppers

In the folk medicine of Utah, Indiana, Illinois, Ohio, and China, cayenne pepper (*Capsicum* spp.) is used in liniments and plasters. Residents of the Southwest use cayenne pepper in their liniments as well. Cayenne became a popular natural remedy thanks to Thomsonian herbalism, which was a well-known herbal movement throughout rural New England and the Midwest in the early 1800s. A constituent of cayenne, called capsaicin, which is also used in pepper spray, stimulates pain receptors without actually burning the tissues. Below is a simple cayenne liniment.

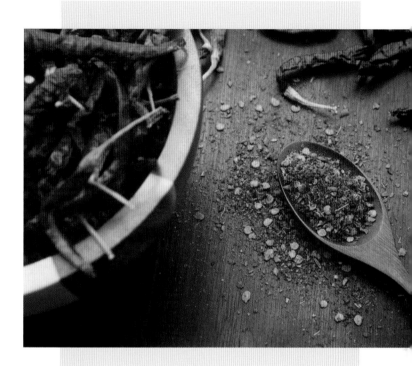

Directions: *Place one ounce of cayenne pepper in a quart of rubbing alcohol. Let the solution stand for two to three weeks, shaking the bottle each day. (You'll need to make this one in advance!) Then, apply to the affected area. (This remedy is not for internal use.)*

A faster alternative is to place one ounce of cayenne pepper in one pint of boiling water. Simmer for half an hour. Do not strain, but add one pint of rubbing alcohol. Let cool to room temperature.

Probably the fastest method, from contemporary North American Chinese folklore, is to gently melt five teaspoons of Vaseline in a pan and add to it one teaspoon of cayenne pepper. Stir well and allow to cool to room temperature. Apply as desired.

Secret Fixes for Eyes, Teeth, and More

Bladder and Kidney

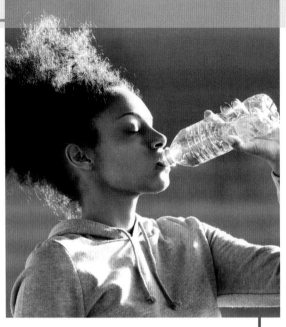

The urinary system includes those organs of the body that produce or eliminate urine. By controlling urine flow, the system maintains proper water balance in the body. Changes in urine and urinary habits that do not seem to have an obvious cause may be symptoms of disease. An accurate diagnosis by a physician is the first step to proper treatment.

Most pathological conditions of the kidney and bladder are not appropriate for self-treatment with natural or home remedies. Even bladder infections, the least serious of common urinary tract conditions, require a diagnosis to rule out sexually transmitted diseases or more serious kidney involvement. Most of the natural remedies below for treating urinary tract infections work in the same way as conventional treatment recommendations, however. For example, drinking adequate water to wash out bacteria is a standard procedure in both folk and conventional medicine for treating urinary tract infections.

Most of the natural remedies in this section use herbs with mild diuretic properties. These herbs increase the flow of urine through the urinary tract, helping to wash out irritating substances. In Germany, the use of such mild diuretics is called "flushing out therapy"; in that country, the therapy is a routine conventional treatment for bladder infections and stone prevention. Research has shown that mild diuretics increase urination and reduce joint swelling. Thus, mild natural diuretics are also used in Germany for treating the swollen joints of arthritis.

An important restriction on the use of herbal diuretics, however, is in cases of edema resulting from heart, kidney, or liver disease. (The condition was once known as "dropsy.") Edema requires careful medical attention—and properly monitored doses of diuretics. Although some natural remedies were once used to treat edema, during the 20th century, modern medical science has discovered safer and more effective treatments for the condition.

The remedies in this section are found in many cultures throughout the world. In fact, most of these remedies would be included in classes on urinary tract herbs in medical schools in Germany, where doctors and pharmacists are required by law to receive training in medical herbalism.

Kidney Stones

A myth perpetuated in many modern herbals and collections of natural remedies is that certain herbs or foods will "dissolve stones." Kidney stones are formed when certain salts become too concentrated in the urine. Once formed, they do not readily dissolve back into the urine, however, and must either pass down the urinary tract or be broken up or dissolved by conventional medical means. Certain individuals, sometimes referred to in conventional medicine as "stone formers," tend to suffer repeat attacks of kidney stones. For them, the best treatment for kidney stones is prevention, which involves drinking plenty of water to dilute the urine. Drinking large amounts of fluids, particularly at night, reduces urine concentration so that stones cannot form.

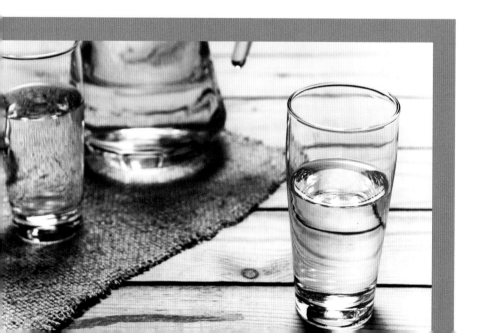

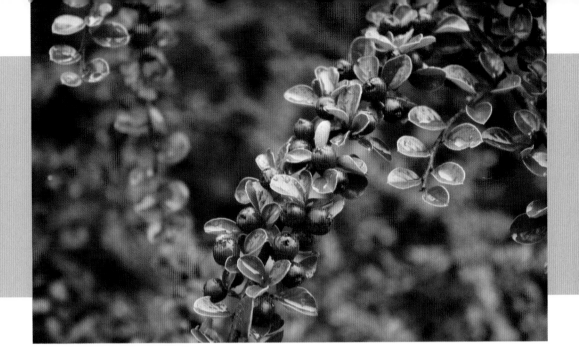

remedies for bladder and kidney issues

Bearberry

The herb bearberry (*Arctostaphylos uva-ursi*), sometimes called uva ursi (bearberry in Latin), was first recorded as a medicinal herb in the 13th century Welsh herbal book *The Physicians of Myddfai*. The berries of the plant are a favorite food of bears—thus its name. Its use as a diuretic and lower urinary tract disinfectant is recorded in subsequent centuries throughout the British Isles and northern Europe.

Bearberry is still one of the most often prescribed urinary tract herbs by professional medical herbalists in North America and Europe, and it is approved in Germany for use by medical doctors in the treatment of bladder infections. Arbutin, a constituent in bearberry, is broken down in the body and transformed into an antimicrobial substance that is excreted in the urine, thus delivering an antibiotic directly to the site of the bladder infection. What's more, animal research in Spain in 1994 demonstrated that bearberry teas could lower the risk factors for kidney stones and kidney infections, although the effect was mild. Avoid using bearberry during pregnancy or lactation.

Directions: *Simmer ½ ounce of bearberry leaves in one pint of water for five minutes. Let steep until the water reaches room temperature. For a bladder infection, strain and drink one ounce three times a day for up to five days.*

Corn Silk

Corn silk (*Zea mays*), the hairy projections from the end of an ear of corn, was introduced as a medicine to the Western world after the European invasion of Mexico, Central America, and South America. Corn, native to those areas, is now cultivated not only in the Americas, but as far away as Africa, India, and China. Corn silk tea was used as a diuretic by American Indians and is now used in the same way in traditions throughout North America and Europe. It has even entered into formal Chinese medical traditions, where it is called yu mi shu. It is often prescribed as a diuretic by professional medical herbalists of Europe, North America, and Australia.

Directions: *Fill a one-quart jar 1/3 full of fresh corn silk. Pour enough boiling water to fill the jar, cover, and let cool to room temperature. Strain and drink the quart in four doses during the day for seven to ten days.*

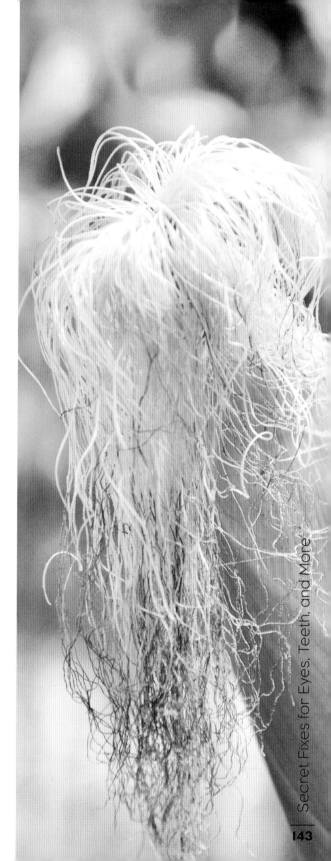

Secret Fixes for Eyes, Teeth, and More

"Joe-Pye" Weed

Queen of the meadow (*Eupatorium purpureum, Eupatorium maculatum*) was used medicinally by eastern Native Americans, including the Cherokee and Mohawk tribes, before the arrival of European colonists. A healer named Joe Pye reportedly used it to treat a group of colonists suffering from typhoid fever, and the survivors of the epidemic named the plant in honor of him—thus, Joe-Pye weed. It is also called "gravel root" because of its prominent use as a treatment for kidney stones. Queen of the meadow was used by Eclectic physicians from about 1848 until the group's demise in the 1940s. The Eclectics preferred Queen of the meadow over some other diuretic plants because of its mild, non-irritating effects. The Electicis believed the herb was effective in treating kidney stones for two reasons—first, because it increased the flow of urine, preventing stone formation or washing out existing stones, and second, it reduced inflammation and pain in the urinary tract.

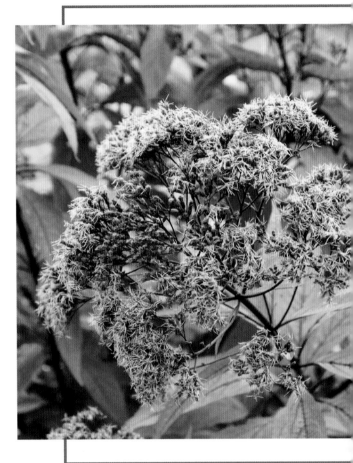

Queen of the meadow is recommended in the remedies of North Carolina residents for treating or preventing painful urinary tract conditions. The plant is still prescribed as a diuretic for bladder infections and kidney stones by professional medicinal herbalists in North America.

Directions: *Add ½ ounce of Queen of the meadow to a pint of water. (Queen of the meadow may be sold in your herb shop under the name "gravel root.") Cover and simmer for twenty minutes. Let cool to room temperature. Drink two to three cups a day, while also drinking plenty of water.*

Goldenrod

If you're not allergic to this common cause of hay fever, goldenrod (*Solidago* spp.) may be as useful to you as a mild diuretic that helps to flush out the urinary tract. It was used for this purpose by the Chippewa tribe; it is used in the same way today in the natural medicine of Indiana. (Goldenrod was also used in Europe as a treatment for wounds—the flowers would be packed into a wound to stop the bleeding.)

Directions: *Place a handful of goldenrod flowers in a one-pint jar and fill with boiling water. Cover and let cool to room temperature. To treat a bladder infection, strain and drink the pint in three doses during the day for seven to ten days.*

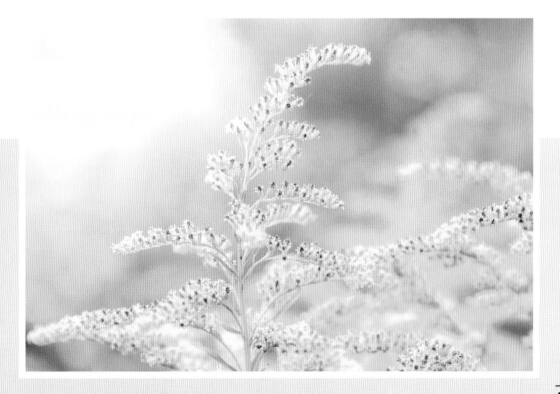

Pumpkin Seeds

Another diuretic often mentioned in natural remedy literature is pumpkin seeds (*Cucurbita pepo*). The medical traditions of New England, Indiana, and Louisiana all suggest taking a few pumpkin seeds to promote urination.

Contemporary German physicians use pumpkin seed preparations to treat difficult urination that accompanies enlarged prostate (when prostate cancer as a cause has been ruled out). Two constituents in pumpkin seeds, adenosine and cucurbitacin, both have diuretic properties.

Directions: Crush a handful of fresh pumpkin seeds and place in the bottom of a one-pint jar. Fill with boiling water. Let cool to room temperature. Strain and drink a pint of the tea each day.

Also, you can eat pumpkin seeds according to taste. It is best to remove the shells and eat them with little or no salt.

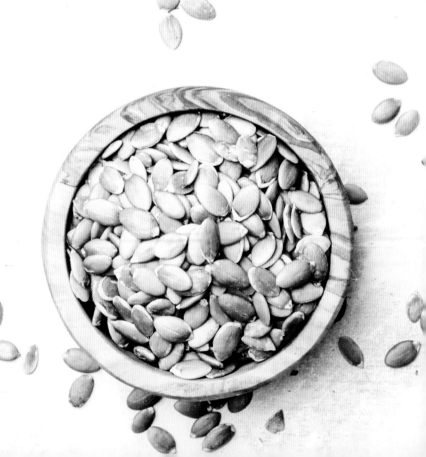

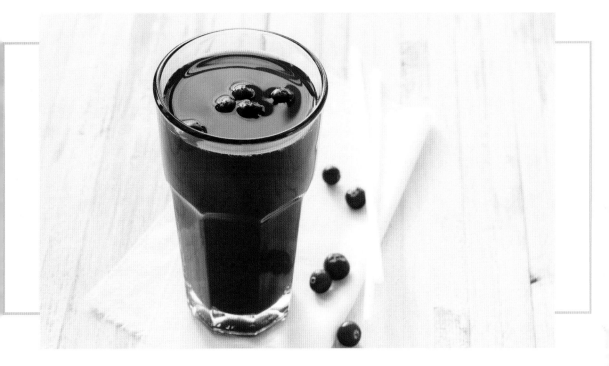

Cranberry Juice

One of the most famous natural remedies for bladder infections—widely followed today throughout North America—is to drink cranberry juice.

This remedy, which has been studied in modern clinical trials, has been found to be effective in preventing, but not treating, bladder infections. A study conducted at the Brigham and Women's Hospital in Boston, and published in the prestigious *The Journal of the American Medical Association,* found that consumption of about twelve ounces of commercial cranberry juice each day for a month reduced bacterial counts in the lower urinary tracts of elderly women. Several other trials have shown similar results. (Using cranberry juice as a preventive may be very useful to bedridden elders, who are at higher risk for bladder infections.)

Constituents in the cranberry juice help to prevent bacteria from sticking to the walls of the urinary tract, making the bacteria easier to flush out. Once the infection is underway, however, and the bacteria have set up shop, the cranberry juice is not of much use.

Directions: *Obtain a sugar-free cranberry juice or juice concentrate from a health food store. (The brands in supermarkets contain enough sugar to depress the activity of the immune system.) Drink eight to twelve ounces of the juice a day to prevent infections.*

Secret Fixes for Eyes, Teeth, and More

Parsley

The ancient Egyptians, Greeks, and Romans all used parsley (*Petroselinum crispum*) as a diuretic. The practice continues today both by the Romani and in the tradition of New England. Parsley, which originated in the eastern Mediterranean region, was introduced to England in the year 1548, and within a hundred years, it was recommended in British medical herbals for use as a diuretic in cases of severe edema (dropsy).

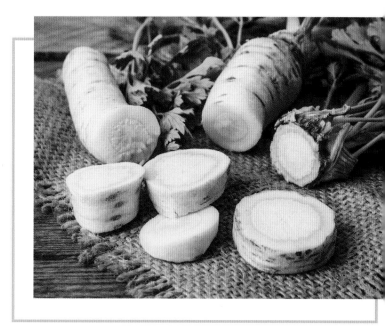

Although edema is now treated with conventional medicine, parsley can still be used to remedy other conditions. Parsley is approved by the German government for use as a mild diuretic and for treatment of bladder infections. For safety's sake, use parsley root rather than parsley seeds, parsley juice, or parsley leaves. (Parsley seeds can stimulate uterine contractions or irritate the kidneys. Parsley juice can also stimulate uterine contractions and should thus be avoided during pregnancy. And, although parsley leaves are nutritious, they do not contain much of the diuretic constituents of the plant.) This formula is a modification of a Romani diuretic formula used for urinary tract infections and kidney stones.

Directions: Take a handful of parsley roots and cut them into small pieces. Place them in one quart of water, bring to a boil, and simmer for ten to fifteen minutes. Remove from the heat and stir in a handful of rose blossoms. Steep, covered, for ten minutes. Strain and drink five to seven cups of the tea during the course of a day for seven to ten days. Do not use it during pregnancy and lactation.

Anise

The Amish use anise seed (*Pimpinella anisum*) as a diuretic. Residents of the Southwest use it the same way—as did the ancient Egyptians and Greeks. The Greek herbalist Dioscorides, whose book of herbal medicine was used by doctors in Europe for at least 1600 years, stated that anise seed "provokes urine." Anise, better known in medical herbalism as a digestive stimulant, is probably one of the mildest diuretics in this section.

Directions: Crush one teaspoon of anise seeds in a grinder or with a mortar and pestle. Place in a cup and fill with boiling water. Cover well, and let steep for ten minutes. Strain and drink two to three cups a day. Don't take anise except as a simple food spice in pregnancy, because anise can stimulate uterine contractions when taking the above dose.

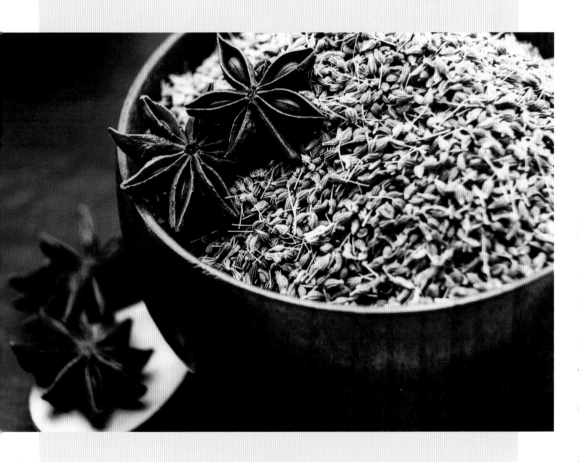

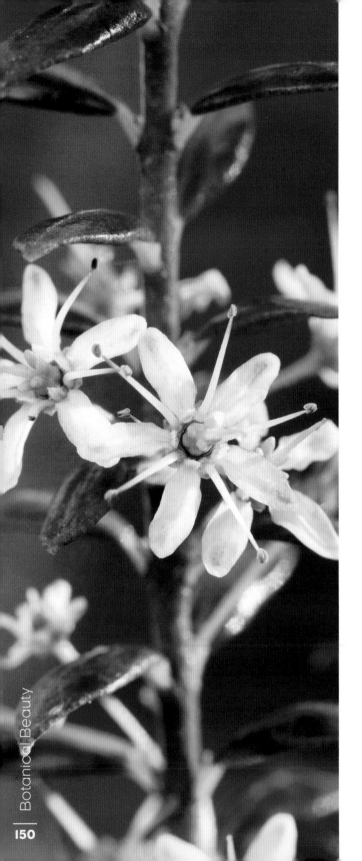

Buchu

The Hottentot tribe of southern Africa first acquainted Europeans with the use of buchu (*Barosma betulina*). In 1821, it was imported to England. By 1840, it appeared in the *United States Pharmacopoeia* as an official medicine. It was used for treating urinary tract infections by all schools of medicine during that period. (The Eclectic physicians cautioned that the plant's oils could further irritate those urinary tract infections that are accompanied by burning or stinging pain, however.) The plant's constituents are probably its aromatic peppermint-like oils.

Directions: Place ½ ounce of buchu leaves and ½ ounce of marshmallow root (Althea officinalis) *in one quart of water. Cover the pot and simmer on the lowest heat for thirty to forty minutes. Allow to cool to room temperature. Strain and drink one-ounce doses three to four times a day for seven to ten days.*

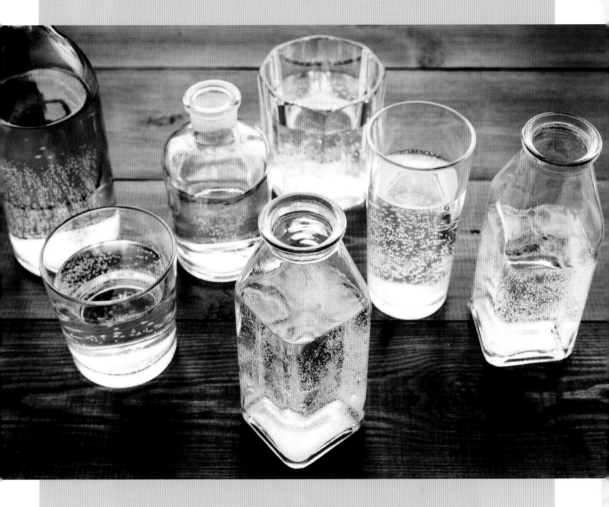

Water

The most obvious diuretic to increase the flow of urine is water. Simply drinking plenty of water—eight glasses a day—can increase urine flow, dilute the urine to prevent stone formation, and wash out bacteria that may cause infections. Some of the benefits of mild diuretic teas used by physicians in Germany and by professional herbalists in North America come from the tea's increased volume of water.

Directions: *Drink eight glasses of water a day. Or, one day a week, drink eight glasses of water in succession, within fifteen minutes, to flush out the urinary tract.*

Cleavers

Cleavers *(Galium aparine)* is most commonly used in contemporary medical herbalism as a "blood cleanser" for skin conditions. But a tea made of cleavers—also known as goosegrass or bed straw (it was also used to stuff mattresses)—has been used as a diuretic as well. The Ojibwa Indians used it or this purpose, as did the physicians of the Physiomedicalist and Eclectic schools.

Directions: *Place one ounce of cleavers in a quart of water and simmer for ten to fifteen minutes. Let cool to room temperature. Drink the quart of tea in three to four divided doses throughout the day.*

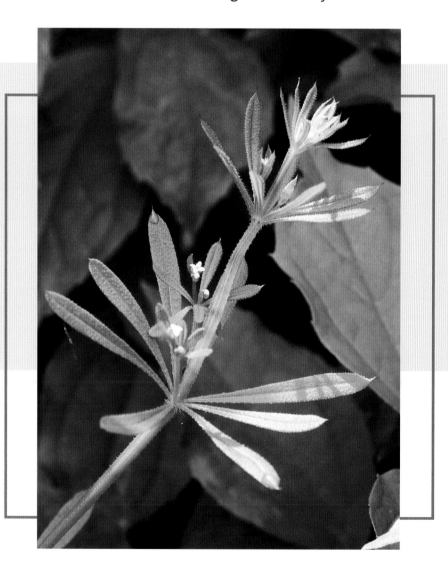

Constipation can mean either difficult or infrequent passage of the feces. Normal healthy bowels will produce between one and three bowel movements a day. Not an illness in itself, constipation, whether chronic or acute, can be the symptom of anything from a low-fiber diet to more serious illnesses. A medical checkup is warranted in any case of severe or persistent constipation. Constipation accompanied by nausea, vomiting, abdominal pain, or rectal bleeding or in the presence of any inflammatory bowel disease should never be treated with laxatives.

The most common cause of constipation in modern society is the modern diet. Constipation is classified by medical anthropologists H.C. Trowell and D.P. Burkitt as a "Western" condition, meaning that the condition does not appear in primitive people eating traditional diets— that is, until Western foods, such as sugar, white flour, and canned goods, are added.

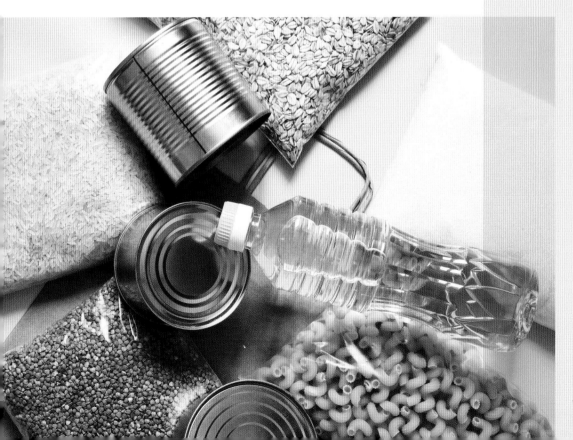

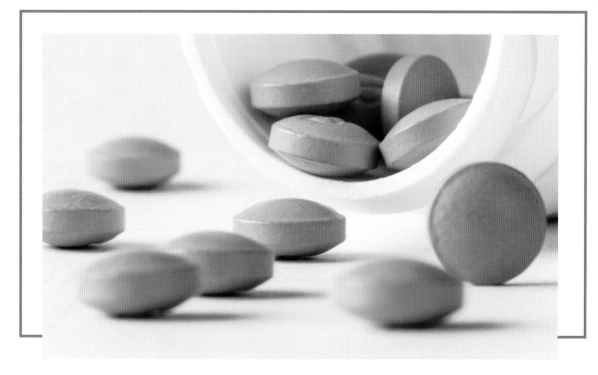

Conventional physicians, alternative doctors, and natural healers alike all warn against the use of strong laxatives to force a bowel movement. From a medical point of view, if the constipation is due to a serious underlying disease, the laxative can cause injury and make that condition worse. Chronic use of strong laxatives also creates "laxative dependence"—a condition in which the bowels become so exhausted that they can no longer provide a normal bowel movement without the stimulation of more laxatives. Laxative dependence can also cause electrolyte (such as sodium and potassium) imbalances.

Conventional treatment for constipation, after a thorough investigation of the cause, is to increase fiber and liquids in the diet and to administer bulk laxatives (also called stool softeners) such as psyllium husks. An increase in fruits and vegetables in the diet is also encouraged. Eat six or more servings of vegetables each day.

Many of the remedies for treating constipation include herbs that act as strong laxatives, but their use for more than seven to ten days is not warranted. Anything stronger than a bulk laxative is contraindicated in pregnancy, however, because the same constituents that make the colon wall contract to produce a bowel movement can make the uterus contract as well. Stimulating laxatives are also contraindicated for use in children under twelve years of age.

remedies for constipation

Senna

Well-known as a laxative, senna leaves (*Cassia senna*), most of which are imported from India, were brought to this country by European colonists. A North American variety of senna was used in the same way by Native Americans in eastern parts of the United States. Senna leaves have been used as a laxative by the Amish. Senna has been used for the same purpose in the natural medicine of New England, Appalachia, and the Southwest.

Senna is also a component of some over-the-counter laxatives in North America and Europe. It is contraindicated in children, during pregnancy, and for more than ten days at a time.

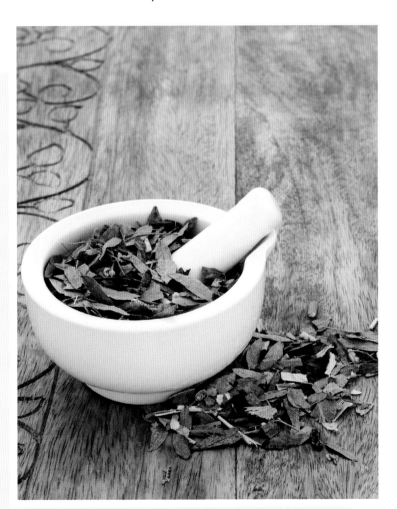

Directions: Do not use excessive amounts of senna. Place ¼ to ½ teaspoon of the dried crushed leaves or powder in a cup and fill with boiling water. Let steep seven to ten minutes. (A full teaspoon in a cup of tea is strong enough to produce abdominal cramping.)

Epsom Salts

Epsom salts are composed of magnesium sulfate. Their use as a commercial laxative spread quickly in the medicine of Europe; the salts remain popular there today. Epsom salts are now produced industrially and not from the springs in Epsom. The salts act as a laxative by drawing water out of the body and into the intestine. Habitual use can cause dehydration and laxative dependence, however, so don't use Epsom salts for more than seven days.

Directions: *Place two or three teaspoons of Epsom salts in a glass of warm water and drink. Do this once a day.*

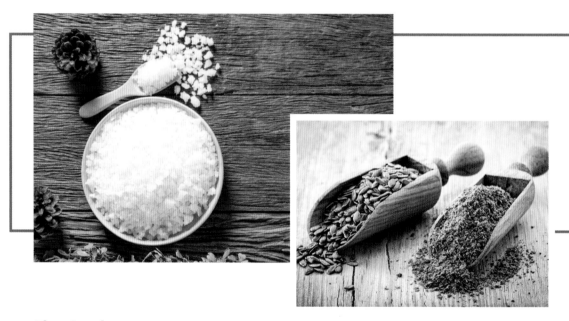

Flax Seeds

Flax seed *(Linum usitatissimum)* is a New England remedy for treating constipation. The remedy is also used among the Amish and by some Romani. Flax is a bulk laxative, meaning that its fiber absorbs water, expands, and provides bulk for bowel movements. Flax seed also contains high amounts of essential fatty acids. Flax seed works in the same way as psyllium seed, the chief component of the bulk laxative Metamucil.

Directions: *Take two teaspoons of flax seeds. Grind them and add to an eight-ounce glass of water. Let stand for half an hour and drink, seeds and all.*

A Romani Formula

The following formula, related in Wanja von Hausen's *Gypsy Folk Medicine*, combines several laxative substances with herbs to reduce tension and improve digestion. Note the absence of any strong laxatives, making it a safe formula for regular use.

Directions: Mix a half-handful of rosemary blossoms or leaves and a handful of black elderberries in a pint of extra virgin olive oil. Shake well and store for three days in a cool, dark place.

Crush one tablespoon of flax seeds in a coffee grinder or with a mortar and pestle. Place the crushed seeds in a bowl, adding the olive oil and herb mixture. Crush two tablespoons of valerian root and add to the mixture. Place the entire mixture in a jar, shake well, and store for seven days, shaking it once or twice a day. Strain the oil through cheesecloth or gauze, and store in a cool, dark place. Take one tablespoon first thing in the morning on an empty stomach. If needed, take a second tablespoon in the evening before dinner. Keep taking the oil until your bowel movements are regular.

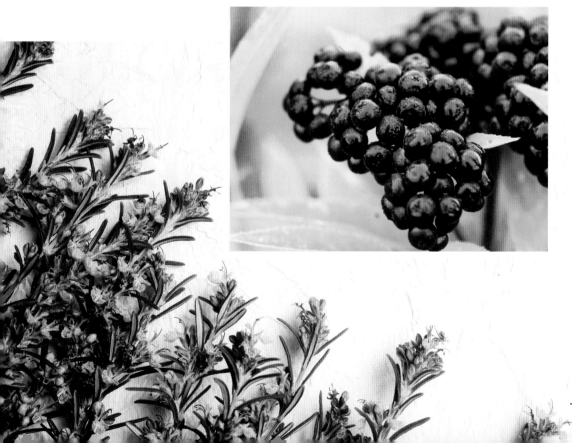

Sesame Seeds

According to the Amish, sesame seeds have a laxative effect. Chinese natural medicine claims the same. The seeds are nutritious and also contain about fifty-five percent oil, which helps to moisten the intestines in those suffering from dry constipation.

Directions: Eat up to ½ ounce of sesame seeds a day. Grind them fresh in a coffee grinder and sprinkle on food like a condiment.

Hot Water

A remedy from New England also mentioned by the Amish is to drink a cup of hot water in the morning. Similar practices, slightly modified, appear throughout the world. In the medicine of India, the prescription is to drink a quart of room temperature water in the morning. German followers of the water cures of Father Sebastian Kneipp take the water hot in one-tablespoon doses every half hour all day.

Drinking water in the morning to produce a bowel movement has a solid psychological basis. An internal digestive reflex causes the bowels to contract and move the stool in the direction of the anus in response to stretching of the stomach. The stretch reflex can be triggered most easily in the morning, when the stomach is most contracted. Drinking water can trigger this stretch reflex.

Directions: Drink one to three cups of hot water first thing in the morning on an empty stomach.

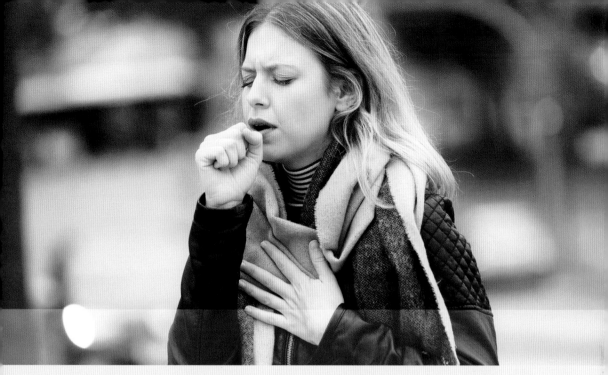

Coughs

Coughing can result from inhaling dust, dirt, or irritating fumes; from breathing icy air; or from mistakenly drawing food into the airways. It can also be caused by mucus and other secretions from such respiratory disorders as the common cold, influenza, pneumonia, or tuberculosis.

The respiratory passages in the throat and lungs are constantly kept moist by a layer of mucus. This mucus traps small particles, viruses, bacteria, dust, pollen, or other materials. The surfaces of these passageways are so sensitive to touch that any irritation there will cause a cough reflex—a reflex that expels the irritating matter at velocities as high as 100 miles per hour. This reflex usually removes any loose mucus or other matter. A cough is thus a healthy healing mechanism, necessary to remove allergens, viruses, bacteria, or foreign matter from the respiratory tract.

Both pharmaceutical drugs and natural remedies aid coughs in several ways. Some remedies, like the herbs licorice or marshmallow, are demulcents; they moisten and soothe the throat and bronchial tract, reducing the cough reflex by reducing irritation of the tissues. Others, such as garlic or honey, are expectorants and work by promoting the secretion of fresh mucus, which aids the body in washing out irritants. Finally, cherry bark and the over-the-counter drug dextromethorphan are respiratory sedatives. They act on the nervous system to reduce the cough reflex. Such a reduction is appropriate for short-term use when an unproductive cough interferes with sleep or is overly-exhausting. Sedatives are not appropriate for productive coughs with a lot of mucus, however, because the cough is necessary to clear the lungs of mucus.

According to the Public Citizen Health Research Group, dextromethorphan is the best cough suppressant to use. It is a component of many over-the-counter cough remedies and syrups. The Public Citizen Health Research Group recommends purchasing generic dextromethorphan at a pharmacy or taking a product containing only dextromethorphan, which will suppress a cough for about twelve hours and allow a good night's sleep.

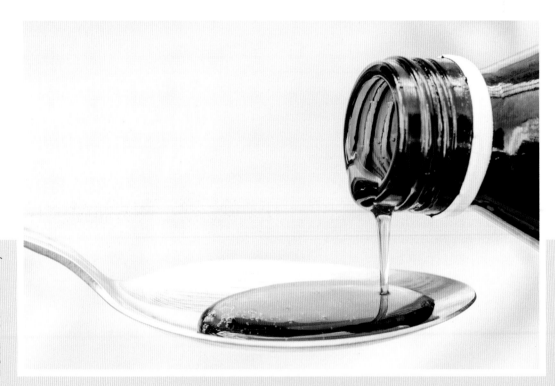

The actions of cough remedies, even the over-the-counter pharmaceutical types, are difficult to prove. There is no scientific evidence supporting that these herbs effectively treat coughs, probably due to the difficulty in accurately measuring expectoration.

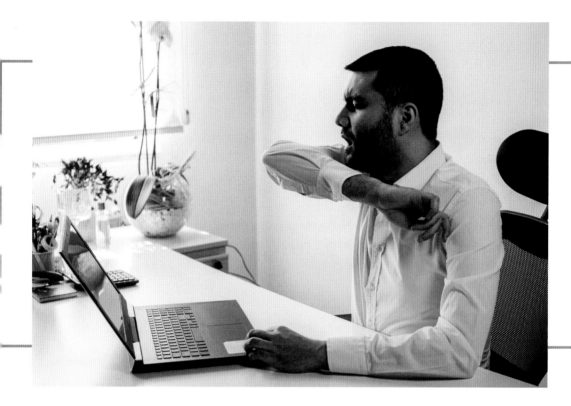

coughs, dry and wet

With some coughs—such as "wet" coughs—plenty of mucus is present, but the mucus is thick, gummy, and hard to expel. Acrid, irritating, and stimulating herbs are helpful for treating these types of coughs because they stimulate the flow of new clean mucus, which helps expel the old.

"Dry" coughs typically accompany the flu. Acrid and stimulating herbs only irritate dry coughs further because there is little mucus to expel. To treat a dry cough, try a soothing herb such as slippery elm, mallow, or licorice.

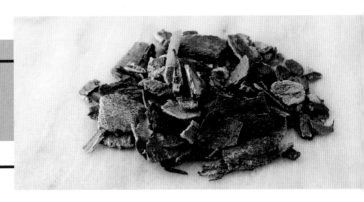

remedies for coughs

Wild Cherry Bark

The use of wild cherry bark (*Prunus serotina*) to treat coughs was taught to the British colonists by the Cherokee and the Iroquois eastern Indian tribes. Use of the bark became very popular throughout the United States in the 19th century. "Wild cherry" cough drops are available in stores today, although they are now made artificial flavors instead of actual wild cherry bark.

The bark's constituent prunasin reduces the cough reflex, so wild cherry is classified as a cough suppressant. Thus, it requires the same cautions as the over-the-counter medication dextromethorphan. Prunasin is a potentially toxic compound. But, if taken as a tea in the correct quantities, adults are safe using it. All cases of toxicity from wild cherry have occurred in children eating the fruit—called "chokecherries"—along with the toxic pits, which contain large amounts of prunasin and related compounds.

Wild cherry has expectorant and demulcent properties, too, so this herb is like a complete cough formula all rolled up into one. Wild cherry bark is especially suited to dry, irritating coughs. Combining it with another demulcent will further improve its effects.

Directions: Place one tablespoon of wild cherry bark and an equal part of licorice root in one pint of water. Boil for five minutes, remove from heat, sweeten with ½ cup of honey. Let stand until the mixture cools to room temperature. The dose is ¼ cup, no more than five times a day. To remain on the side of caution, don't give cherry bark to children under the age of twelve. Adults shouldn't take cherry bark for more than three consecutive days. Women should avoid cherry bark if they are pregnant or nursing.

Flax Seed

New Englanders and residents of other eastern states use boiled flax seeds *(Linum usitatissimum)* to treat coughs. Boiled flax seeds make a thick demulcent that is soothing to the throat and bronchial tract.

Directions: Boil two or three tablespoons of flax seeds in one cup of water for a few minutes, until the water becomes gooey. Strain. Add equal parts of honey and lemon juice. For a dry irritable cough that's not producing much mucus, take one-tablespoon doses as needed.

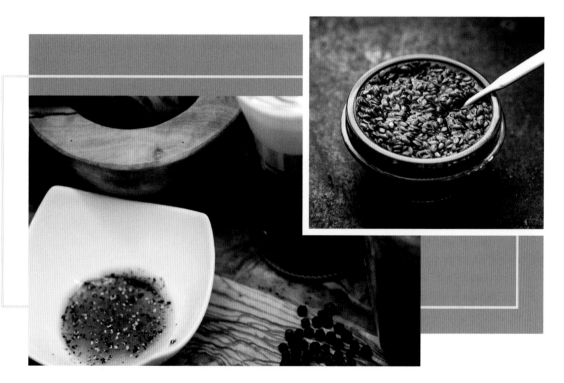

Black Pepper

A remedy for coughs from New England, which also appears in Chinese folk medicine, is black pepper *(Piper nigrum)*. The irritating properties of black pepper stimulate circulation and the flow of mucus. Black pepper works best on coughs producing a thick mucus; it is inappropriate for a dry, irritable cough with little expectoration.

Directions: Place one teaspoon of black pepper and one tablespoon of honey in a cup and fill with boiling water. Let steep for ten to fifteen minutes. Take small sips as needed.

Horehound

A remedy for coughs from contemporary New Mexico is horehound (*Marrubium vulgare*), a European plant that arrived in North America with both the Spanish and northern European colonists. Horehound has been used to treat coughs in European medicine since the time of the ancient Greeks. It was an official cough remedy in the *United States Pharmacopoeia* between 1840 and 1910.

Horehound stimulates the flow of mucus, and is indicated for use in moist unproductive coughs. It can be irritating and increase the discomfort of dry coughs, however.

Directions: *Place one tablespoon of dried horehound in a cup and fill with boiling water. Cover and let steep for fifteen minutes. Sweeten with honey. Drink in 1/2-cup doses as often as desired.*

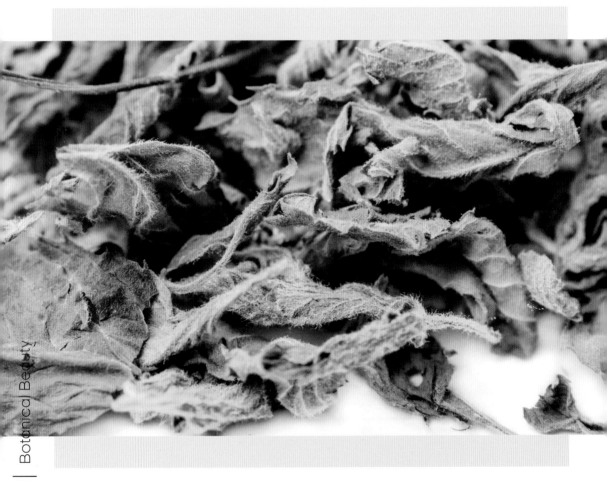

Mustard Seed

An old New England cough remedy calls for mustard seed. Mustard is also used for treating coughs in the medicine of China. Mustard has irritating sulfur-containing compounds that stimulate the flow of mucus. Like pepper, above, it is only appropriate for congested productive coughs with plenty of mucus present. It will irritate a dry cough and make it worse.

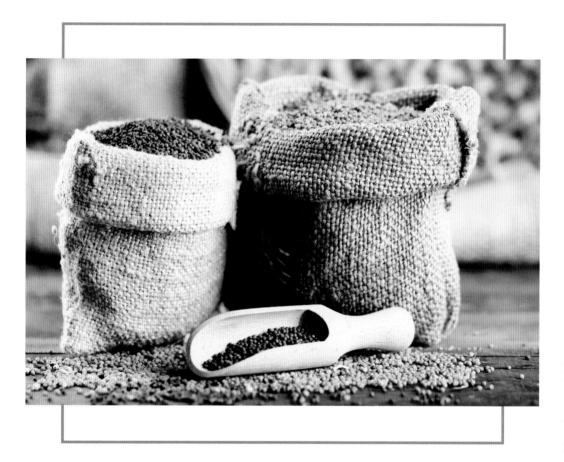

Directions: Crush one teaspoon of mustard seeds or grind them in a coffee grinder. Place the seeds in a cup and fill with warm water. Steep for fifteen minutes. (The expectorant compounds are not released until the mustard seeds are crushed or broken and allowed to sit in water or some other medium for about fifteen minutes.) Take in ¼-cup doses throughout the day.

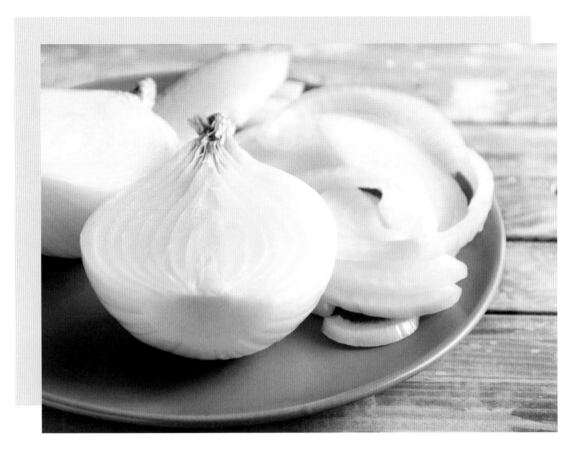

Onion Syrup

In *American Folk Medicine*, folklorist Clarence Meyer suggests taking a honey-and-onion syrup for treating coughs. Onions have anti-inflammatory properties that may reduce throat irritation, and honey is a natural expectorant, promoting the free flow of mucus. Onions also contain the antiviral constituent protocatechuic acid, which attacks viruses, including the one that may be causing the cough.

Directions: *Chop six white onions and place them in a double boiler. Add ½ cup of honey and the juice of one lemon and cook at lowest heat possible for several hours. Strain the mixture and take by the tablespoon as needed—from every half an hour to every few hours.*

Osha Syrup

Osha *(Ligusticum porteri)* is a medicinal plant popular in the higher elevations of the Rocky Mountains. It has a hot acrid taste, and its constituents possess both expectorant and antiviral properties.

Directions: *Grind one ounce of osha root in a coffee grinder. Heat one pint of honey in a pot, and add the osha root. Simmer slowly until the honey becomes thick. Leave the root in the honey and let cool to room temperature. Do not strain. Take one-tablespoon doses of the syrup four to six times a day as desired.*

Licorice

Licorice root *(Glycyrrhiza glabra)* has been used to treat coughs and bronchial problems in many traditions throughout the world. It is listed in several 19th century medicinal remedy collections from the eastern United States. It was an official medicine in the *United States Pharmacopoeia* from 1820 until 1975; it was recommended as a flavoring agent and a demulcent and expectorant for cough syrups.

Directions: *Slice one ounce of licorice sticks, and add to one quart of boiling water. Steep for twenty-four hours. Drink throughout the day, adding honey to taste.*

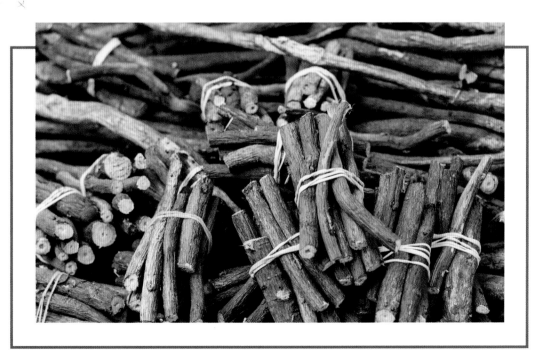

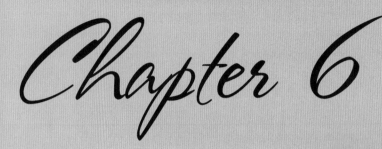

Chapter 6

SOAPS, BALMS, SCRUBS, AND MORE

Explore the following soaps, balms, and scrubs and discover more botanical secrets.

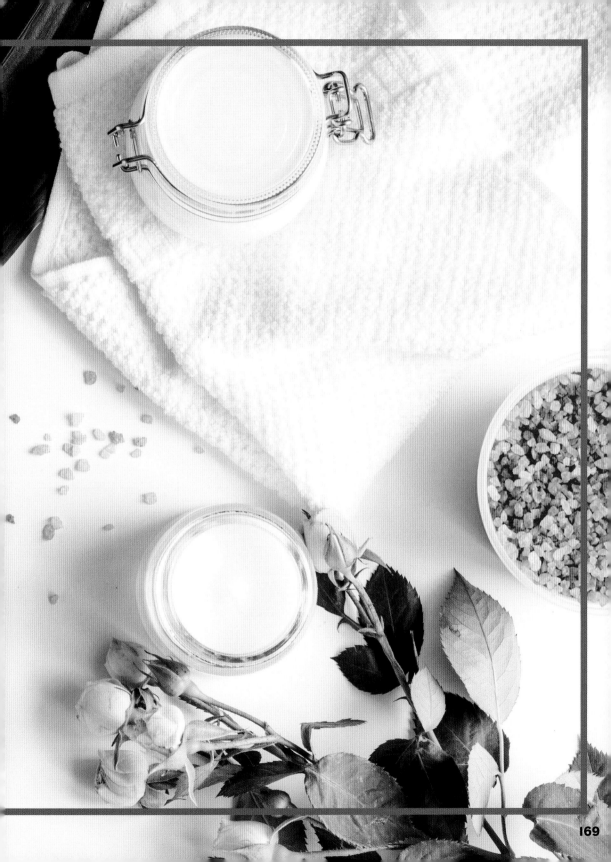

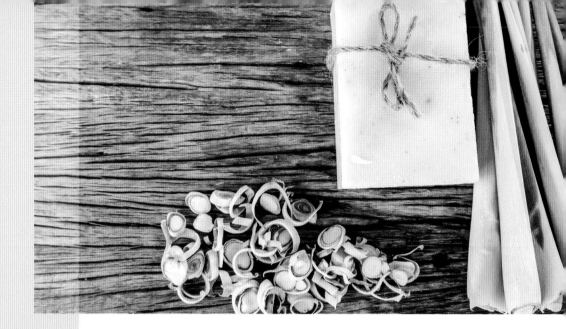

lemongrass soap

- *1/2 gallon cardboard milk or orange juice carton, empty, rinsed, and dried*
- *1/2 pound white vegetable soap compound*
- *2 teaspoons finely minced dried or fresh lemongrass stalk*
- *2-3 drops lemongrass oil*

Directions: *Measure 2 inches up from the bottom of the milk carton. Using a serrated knife or scissors, cut off the bottom of the carton and reserve. Break or cut soap compounds into 1-inch cubes. Place into a 1-quart microwave safe glass measuring cup. Microwave on high in 20-second intervals or less, stirring the soap in between intervals, until the compound melts. Remove the microwave and stir in the lemongrass and essential oil (stir gently to avoid creating bubbles).*

Pour the mixture into the carton and let cool for 10-15 minutes. Use a toothpick or bamboo skewer to distribute lemongrass in the compound, if needed. Place mold in the refrigerator for 1 hour. Turn the soap out and cut into cubes.

orange blossom liquid soap

- Grated peel of 1 lemon
- Grated peel of 1 orange
- 1 cup liquid bubble bath base
- 1/4 teaspoon orange blossom (neroli) oil

Directions: Combine lemon peel, orange peel and 1 cup water in a small saucepan. Simmer for 5 minutes. Remove from heat. Set aside to steep for 1 hour. Insert funnel into a 16-ounce clear bottle with a tight-fitting cap. Place a small coffee filter in the funnel. Pour lemon/orange mixture into the bottle. Discard the filter and add the bubble bath base and essential oil. Seal the bottle tightly and shake well.

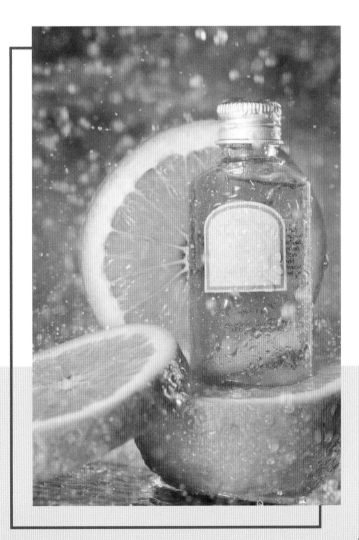

lavender-scented liquid soap

- 1 cup liquid bubble bath base
- 3/4 cup distilled water
- 1/4 teaspoon lavender oil
- 8-10 drops purple soap coloring

Directions: *Combine bubble bath base, distilled water, essential oil, and coloring in a 2-cup measuring cup. Stir well. Insert funnel into a 16-ounce clear bottle with a tight-fitting cap. Pour in mixture.*

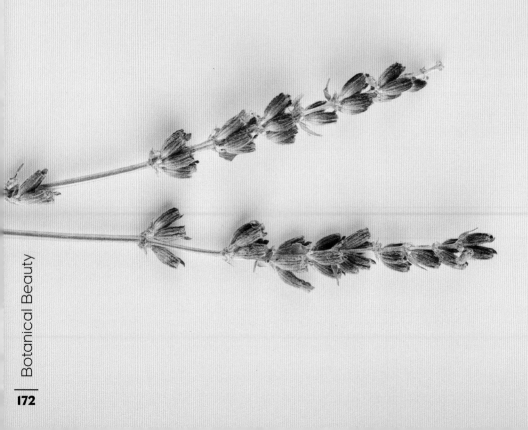

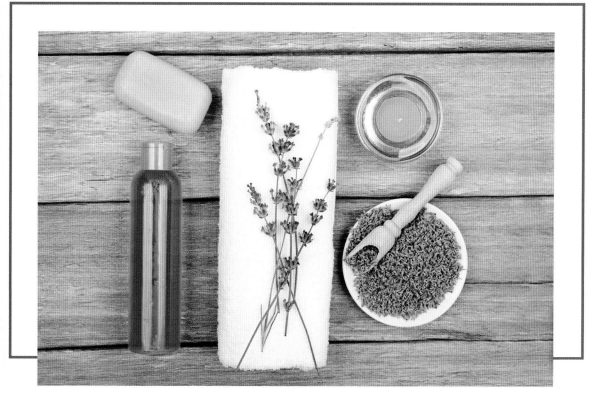

lavender soap

- 1 bar unscented white soap
- 15 drops lavender essential oil
- 5 drops rose essential oil
- 8-10 drops violet or purple soap coloring
- 1/4 cup distilled water
- 1/4 cup dried lavender buds or blossoms

Directions: *Grate soap into medium bowl with a cheese grater. Add essential oils and soap coloring. Add the hot water and stir vigorously to distribute color evenly. Mixture will be the consistency of wet dough. Working quickly, knead in the lavender buds before the soap firms up. Form soap into 3 small balls or oval bars. Set aside on plastic wrap to dry at room temperature 24 hours.*

Soaps, Balms, Scrubs, and More

almond and tangerine glycerin facial soap

- 12 ounces clear or white glycerin soap base
- 1/2 cup ground raw almonds
- 1 tablespoon honey
- 15 drops tangerine or orange oil
- Sunflower oil

Directions: *Lightly grease 6 muffin cups with sunflower oil. Set aside. Slice soap base into slivers. Place in a microwave-safe bowl. Cover loosely with plastic wrap. Microwave on high in 20-second intervals, stirring the soap in between intervals, until the soap is liquid. Stir in almonds, honey, and tangerine oil.*

Quickly pour mixture into muffin cups, filling about 3/4 full. Set aside to firm up, about 1 hour. Run a small knife around the inside edge of the muffin cups to release soap.

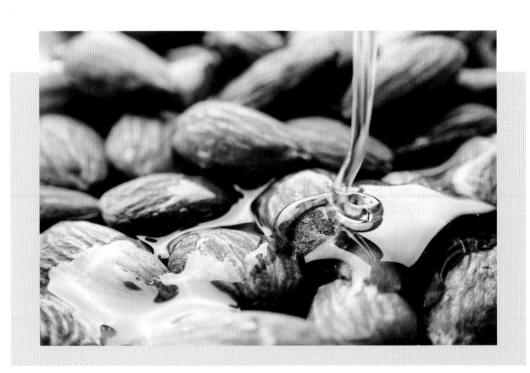

pink himalayan salt grapefruit soap

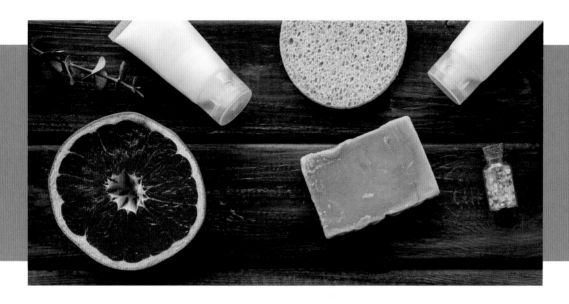

- *1 pound goat's milk soap base*
- *1/4 cup ground pink Himalayan salt*
- *10-15 drops of grapefruit oil*
- *Soap molds*
- *Coconut oil*

Directions: *Prepare the soap molds by lightly greasing with coconut oil. Cut the soap base into chunks, and then melt in a double boiler. (The soap base can also be melted in the microwave: place chunks in a glass bowl, and microwave for 30 seconds. Stir, then microwave for 10 to 20 more seconds, until the base has melted completely.) Remove from heat and add grapefruit essential oil. Stir in salt, and pour mixture into molds. Allow soap to set for at least two hours before removing from molds.*

A perfect soap to use in your morning shower, this pink Himalayan salt grapefruit soap has the familiar, citrusy scent of grapefruit to wake up your mind and uplift your mood. Pink Himalayan salt is said to detoxify the skin and balance pH, while also acting as an exfoliator. Your skin will be smooth and clean, and your shower will smell delicious!

Soaps, Balms, Scrubs, and More

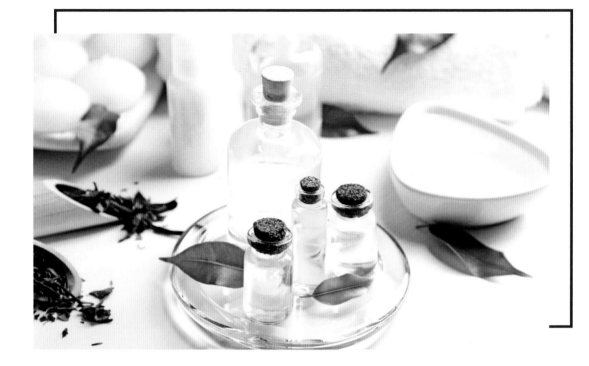

tea tree oil antiseptic soap

- *2 cups clear glycerin soap base*
- *2 tbsp tea tree oil*
- *Soap molds*
- *Coconut oil*

Directions: *Prepare the soap molds by lightly greasing with coconut oil. Cut glycerin soap base into chunks, and then melt in a double boiler or in the microwave (heating for 20-second intervals and stirring the soap in between intervals). Remove from heat, and stir in tea tree oil. Pour into molds, and allow to set for at least two hours.*

Tea tree oil is well renowned for its antibacterial, antifungal, and antiviral properties, making this easy, do-it-yourself soap a must-have for the cold and flu season. It's also excellent to have on hand to wash cuts and scrapes and protect against infection, and to soothe eczema, psoriasis, and other skin conditions. The scent is a bit medicinal, but inhaling the aroma of tea tree has also been shown to ease coughs and congestion. With all of its healthy benefits, this is a useful soap to keep in your medicine cabinet!

elemi and lemon foaming hand soap

- 1 cup distilled water
- 4 drops of elemi oil
- 4 drops of lemon oil
- 1 tbsp unscented Castile soap
- Refillable foaming hand soap dispenser

Directions: *Add distilled water and essential oils to the foaming hand soap dispenser, then add the Castile soap. Screw on the top of the dispenser and swirl to combine.*

Next time you run out of store-bought foaming hand soap, don't run to the grocery store to buy more: save the empty bottle and make your own homemade version! Elemi and lemon essential oils come together to create a bright, uplifting scent, perfect for a morning aromatherapy wake-up. This is also a great soap to keep on hand in the kitchen. Elemi and lemon are both known for their antiseptic properties, so this soap will keep your hands clean while you're preparing food. And who wants fingers that smell like garlic and onions? The oils in this soap help deodorize, leaving behind a sunshiny scent!

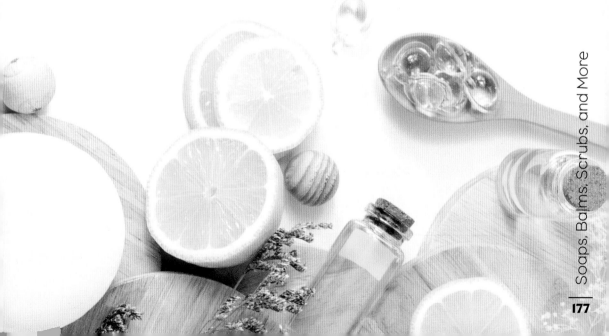

festive exfoliating soap

- 6 ounces shea butter soap base
- 2 tsp oats
- 7 drops cinnamon oil
- 7 drops mandarin oil
- Soap molds
- Coconut oil

Directions: Prepare the soap molds by lightly greasing with coconut oil. Cut shea butter soap base into chunks, and then melt in a double boiler or in the microwave (heating for 20-second intervals and stirring the soap in between intervals). Remove from heat, add oats and essential oils, and stir. Pour into molds, and allow to set for at least two hours.

The spicy scent of cinnamon and the sweet aroma of mandarin have long been associated with the holidays. This warm and brightly scented soap can make you feel festive any time of year! Cinnamon essential oil increases circulation and decreases inflammation in the skin, while mandarin has a calming, uplifting scent that has been shown to reduce anxiety and even nausea. And both oils help diminish skin conditions like acne and rashes. Last but not least, this soap receives some extra oomph from the addition of oats, providing gentle exfoliation.

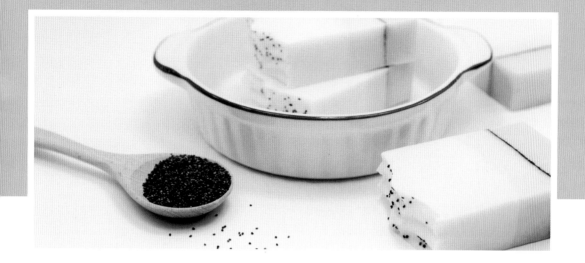

ylang ylang and bergamot exfoliating soap

- 1 pound shea butter soap base
- 15 drops ylang ylang oil
- 10 drops bergamot oil
- 2 tbsp poppy seeds
- Soap molds
- Coconut oil

Directions: *Prepare soap molds by greasing with coconut oil. Cut soap base into chunks, and melt in a double boiler or in the microwave (heating for 20-second intervals and stirring the soap in between intervals). Remove from heat, and stir in essential oils. Allow the mixture to cool slightly before stirring in the poppy seeds—this will ensure that they are evenly distributed throughout the soap, and don't sink to the bottom. Pour mixture into molds, and allow to set for at least two hours.*

As the primary scent used in the famous perfume Chanel No. 5, ylang ylang has long been prized for its rich, floral scent. When it's combined with the citrusy smell of bergamot, it's perfect for creating this lovely bath soap. Not only does it smell good, but it has good-for-you benefits, as well. Ylang ylang helps prevent the signs of aging in skin, while bergamot's antiseptic properties help it fight acne and skin conditions. Poppy seeds provide natural, gentle exfoliation.

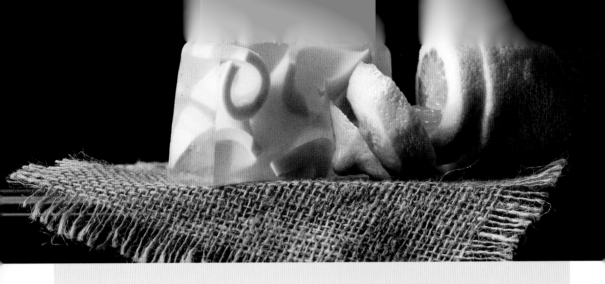

lemon rosemary glycerin soap

- 1 pound clear glycerin soap base
- 15 drops lemon oil
- 15 drops rosemary oil
- Dried lemon peel
- Dried rosemary
- Soap molds
- Coconut oil

Directions: Prepare soap molds by greasing with coconut oil. Cut soap base into chunks, and melt in a double boiler or in the microwave (heating for 20-second intervals and stirring the soap in between intervals). Remove from heat and stir in essential oils. Place lemon peel and rosemary into soap molds, and then fill molds with soap mixture. Allow soap to set for at least two hours. Because this soap contains dried fruit and herbs, use it in a few months to prevent mold.

These soaps are as pretty as they are useful! The clear glycerin provides a versatile base for adding your own fruits and herbs. Experiment with your favorite essential oils and add-ins—try dried flower petals, tea leaves, eucalyptus, or juniper berries. This soap makes a great gift, too!

travel-size refreshing body wash

- 3 1/2 tbsp unscented shower gel base
- 2 drops peppermint oil
- 1 drop rosemary oil
- 1/2 tsp jojoba oil
- 1/2 tsp vitamin E oil
- 2 ounce bottle

Directions: Place all ingredients into a bottle, and swirl to combine. That's it!

This TSA-approved travel-size body wash will help you perk up after a long day of travel. Peppermint essential oil boosts energy and sharpens focus, while rosemary relieves stress and soothes the skin. The addition of skin-loving jojoba oil and vitamin E helps moisturize and nourish with antioxidants. This body wash doesn't lather as much as a store-bought brand, but most commercial soaps add harsh chemicals to create lather. Remember that lather does not necessarily equal clean.

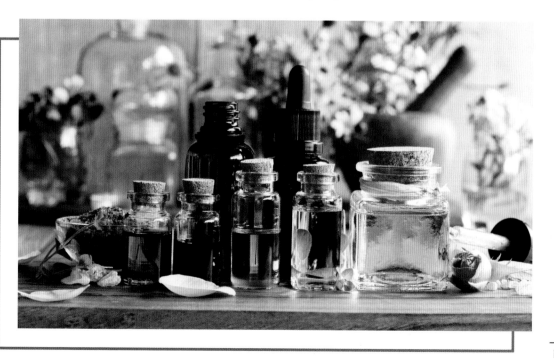

Soaps, Balms, Scrubs, and More

customizable melt and pour soap

- *1/4 cup water*
- *1/4 cup dried and crushed herbs (try lavender, lemon balm, or mint)*
- *6 drops of essential oil (your choice)*
- *2 cups of shredded Ivory soap*
- *Soap molds (optional)*

Directions: *Place shredded Ivory soap in a mixing bowl. In a small pan, add water, herbs, and essential oil and bring to a boil, stirring frequently. Pour the mixture over the Ivory soap and mix well, then let the soap stand for 20 minutes. When it is cool enough, divide the mixture into balls, or press into a soap mold. Once the soap has set, remove from molds, place on a glass plate, and allow to dry for at least 24 hours.*

If you don't have a melt and pour soap base, this versatile recipe lets you use the soap you probably already have in your home! You can use a cheese grater or even a food processor to shred your soap bars, and then use your imagination for your herb and oil additions. Need a soap bar for a relaxing bath? Try dried lavender with chamomile essential oil. Looking for a gentle antiseptic soap to help with acne, eczema, or dermatitis? Dried rosemary with rosemary essential oil might work for you. Mix and match until you find your perfect soap!

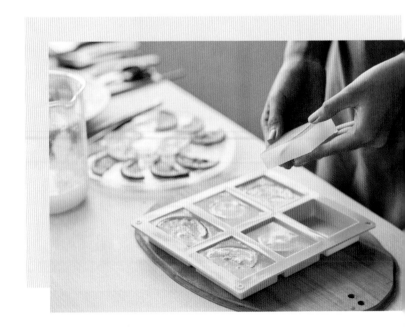

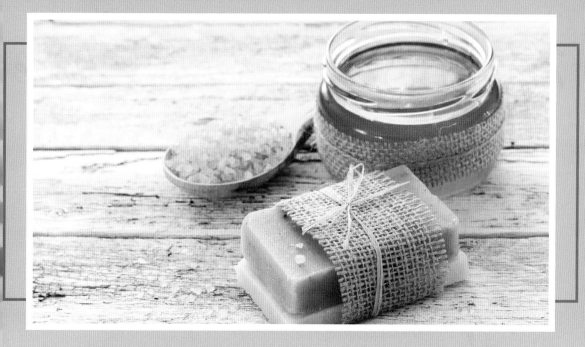

moroccan spiced honey soap

- 1 pound honey soap base
- 6 drops allspice oil
- 6 drops cardamom oil
- 6 drops cinnamon oil
- 6 drops clove essential oil
- Dried bay leaves
- Soap molds
- Coconut oil

Directions: Grease soap molds with coconut oil. Cut soap base into chunks, and melt in a double boiler or in the microwave (heating for 20-second intervals and stirring the soap in between intervals). Remove from heat and mix in all essential oils. Place a bay leaf in each mold, and fill with mixture. Allow to set for two hours before removing from molds.

With its bay leaf accent, this soap is pretty enough to place in a guest bathroom. Allspice, cardamom, cinnamon, and clove essential oils team up to provide a spicy scent and plenty of antiseptic and antioxidant benefits. Look for a melt and pour soap base with honey, which is a natural humectant and helps skin retain moisture.

Soaps, Balms, Scrubs, and More

Balms, Scrubs, and More

coocnut body scrub

- 1/4 to 1/2 cup granulated sugar or coarse salt
- 1/2 cup coconut oil
- Essential oil (citrus or herbal, such as lemon or rosemary), is optional

Directions: Combine granulated sugar, coarse salt or combination of sugar and salt with coconut oil. Do not heat to melt the coconut oil.

Add a few drops of essential oil if desired; blend ingredients well. Place into sanitized, dry container.

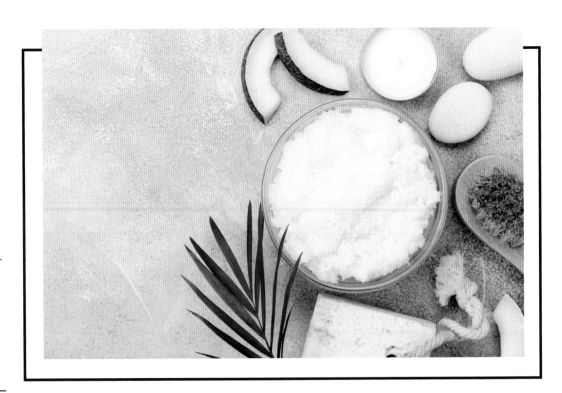

coconut oil salve

- *2 to 3 cups coconut oil*
- *8 to 10 ounces dried herbs (such as calendula, comfrey, rosemary, or yarrow)*
- *1 ounce beeswax per 8 ounces herbal oil*
- *Essential oil (such as lavender, lemon, Roman chamomile or tea tree)*

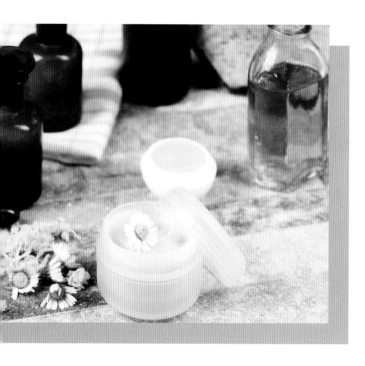

Directions: *Add coconut oil to the upper pot of a double boiler. Sprinkle dried herbs over coconut oil. Add water to the bottom pot of the double boiler; heat to just before simmer.*

Place the pot of coconut oil/herb mixture over the pot of heated water; heat until mixture melts, is unified in color, and the herbs are no longer dry. Remove from heat and cool.

Drain coconut oil from herbs by slowly pouring through a cheesecloth-lined strainer into a medium bowl. Repeat with any remaining oil and herbs if needed.

Carefully wring contents of cooled cheesecloth and herbs into the bowl until no longer residue. Dispose of any remaining dried herbs and cheesecloth.

Add one-ounce beeswax per eight-ounces herb-infused oil back into the upper pot of the double boiler. Reheat water in the lower pot of the double boiler just before simmer. Upon melting, add a few drops of essential oils to the mixture. Mix well; set aside to fully cool. Once cooled, pour the herbal mixture into clean, sanitized containers.

Soaps, Balms, Scrubs, and More

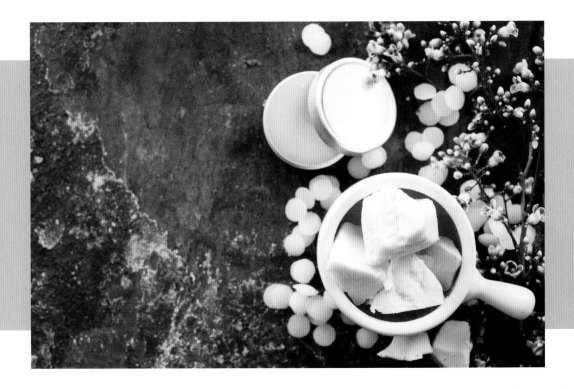

coconut lip balm

- *2 ounces coconut oil*
- *2 ounce clean, sterilized, dry container*
- *Microwave bowl*
- *Clean spoon for mixing*
- *Additional flavored or unflavored oil, if desired (argan, avocado, jojoba, or olive)*
- *Lipstick, if desired*

Directions: *Place coconut oil and a few drops of additional flavored or non-flavored oil (if desired) into a microwavable bowl. Mix well with spoon until smooth consistency. Add a few shavings from the lipstick tube, if desired. Microwave about 10 to 30 seconds depending upon microwave setting until mixture melts.*

Remove from the microwave; blend again with a spoon. When cool, place in the refrigerator to harden. Keep cool; warm with fingertips to apply.

coconut deodorant

- 1/4 cup baking soda
- 1/2 cup arrowroot or cornstarch
- Essential oil (such as lavender, lemon, rosemary, or thyme) if desired
- 6 tablespoons coconut oil
- Sterilized, dry glass jar with lid

Directions: Blend baking soda and arrowroot or cornstarch in a medium-sized bowl. Add a few drops of essential oil, if desired. Add coconut oil; blend with the back of the spoon until well blended. Store in a sterilized glass jar in a cool location.

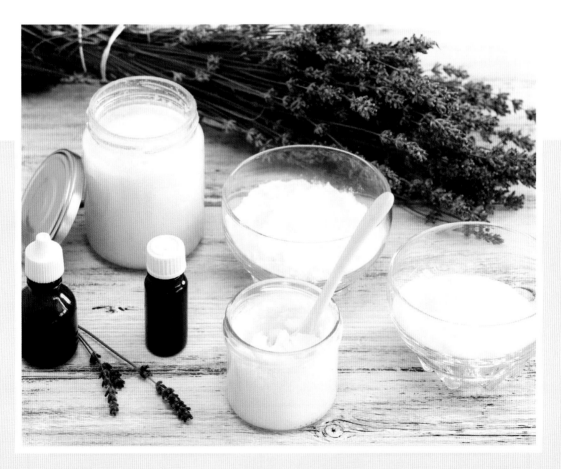

uplifting formula

- *6 drops bergamot oil*
- *3 drops petitgrain oil*
- *3 drops geranium oil*
- *1 drop neroli*
- *2 ounces vegetable oil*

Directions: *Combine all the ingredients. Use as a massage oil, add 1 or 2 teaspoons to your bath, or add 1 teaspoon to a foot bath. For an equally uplifting room or facial spritzer, substitute the same amount of water for the vegetable oil in this formula. Put the water formula in a spray bottle, and spritz or sniff throughout the day as needed.*

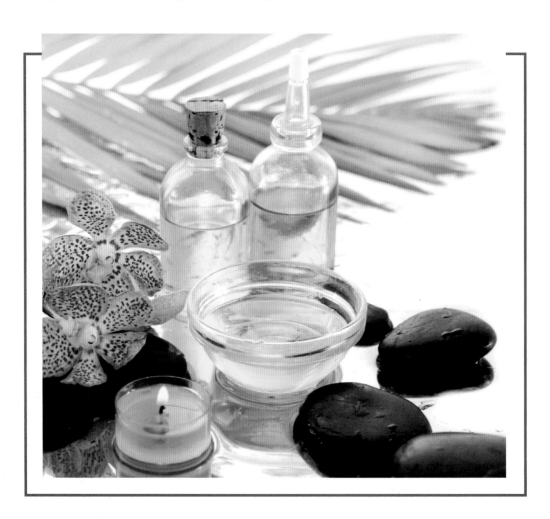

Revitalize Your Hair

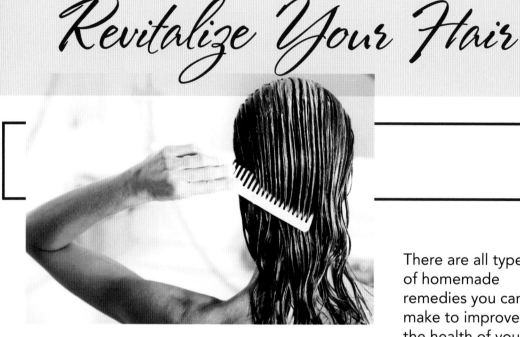

There are all types of homemade remedies you can make to improve the health of your hair. Many store-bought products can contain many harmful chemicals that do more harm to your hair than good. Below are a few useful remedies you can use to replace those damaging products you spend too much money on.

Hair Remedies

- Eggs make a great conditioner: Beat 1 egg white until it's foamy, then stir it into 5 tablespoons of plain yogurt. Apply to your hair section by section; let sit for 15 minutes. Rinse and shampoo as usual.
- Give your hair a conditioning treatment that will leave you feeling like you've been to an expensive salon. Mix 3 eggs, 2 tablespoons extra virgin olive oil, and 1 teaspoon distilled white vinegar. Apply to hair and cover with a plastic cap. Leave on for 30 minutes, then rinse and shampoo as usual.
- Use 1 tablespoon apple cider vinegar mixed with 1 gallon water as an after-shampoo rinse to minimize gray in your hair.
- Before shampooing, briefly soak hair in a small basin of water with 1/4 cup apple cider vinegar added. Repeat several times a week to help control dandruff and remove buildup from sprays, shampoos, and conditioners.

Soaps, Balms, Scrubs, and More

Lice, Your Hair, and Your Health

Lice are wingless insects that live externally on warm-blooded hosts that include every species of bird and mammal. In number, lice are called louse and their eggs are called nits that hatch into nymphs.

Lice favor clean hair and scalp so that they can freely move throughout the hair and their nits can create strong bonds to the hair strands. Lice are contagious, irritating, and are often difficult to remove; however, lice generally do not spread disease. If the scalp is scratched and then inflamed, infection may develop.

Lice can only live off of the human scalp a short amount of time since their only food source is human blood. They cannot live on any other species but they can reside on bed linens, carpets, and furniture—that's why it is important to do a thorough cleaning after lice infestation.

Different types of oils have been used around the world for centuries to treat lice. While coconut oil may not kill lice, it may temporarily immobilize and suffocate them. The viscous consistency of coconut oil is sometimes effective in killing adult lice, but it may be ineffective in killing nits or baby louse. In order for the nits to die they must be manually removed from the strands of hair where they have infiltrated.

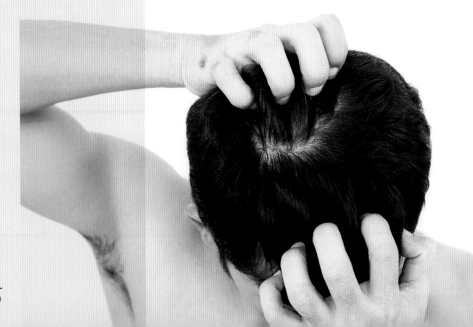

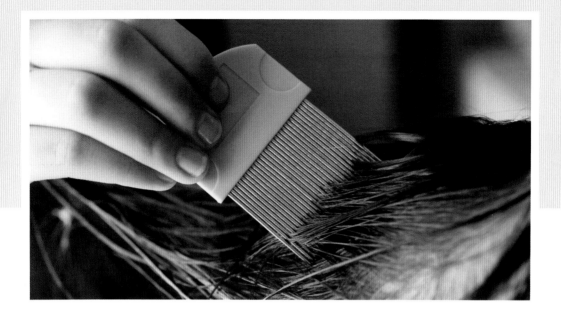

lice-be-gone natural treatment

A natural treatment for lice infestation is as follows:

- *Rinse the scalp with apple vinegar.*
- *Let the apple cider vinegar remain on the hair to dry.*
- *Carefully comb the hair while removing as many nits as possible.*
- *Mix a combination of one cup of coconut oil and 1 to 3 tablespoons of essential oils (such as anise or ylang-ylang with their antibacterial and antifungal properties).*
- *Apply this mixture to the hair and scalp.*
- *Cover the hair and scalp with a thin shower cap or wrap and allow it to set for 12 or more hours, if possible.*
- *The hair should then be shampooed, rinsed, and combed with a special lice comb that has small teeth to remove as many nits and eggs as are visible.*
- *This process can be repeated until the lice are eliminated.*

Soaps, Balms, Scrubs, and More

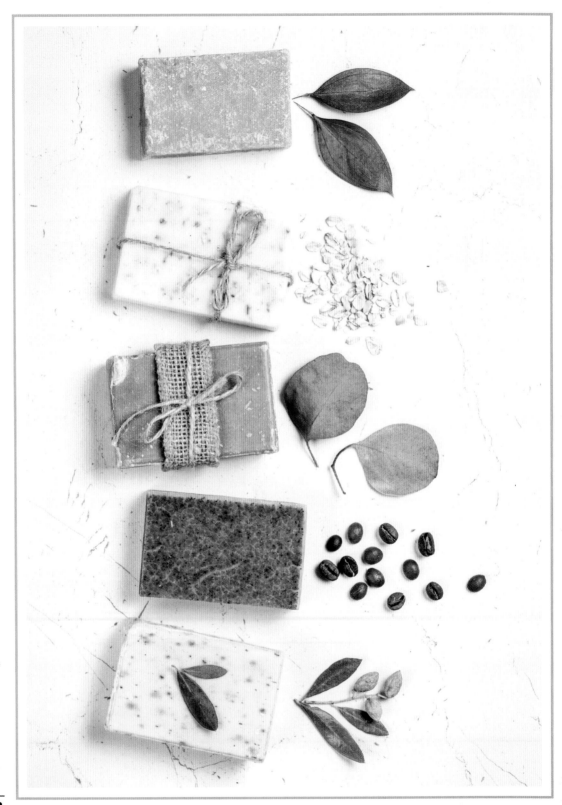